THE E FACTOR

Engage, Energize, Enrich

3 Steps to Vibrant Health

Michelle Robin, D.C.

The E Factor: Engage, Energize, Enrich

First Edition 2012

Cover design: Zachary Cole

Interior design: Rebecca Korphage

ISBN-13: 978-1475196092
ISBN-10: 1475196091

This book is dedicated to all those who believe that wellness
is more than the absence of disease; those who believe it is
the conscious choices that make the most of our human experience,
benefiting self, others and the world.

CONTENTS

FOREWORD

I've known Michelle Robin for twelve years, first as a client, and then as my own wellness caregiver. We have also been colleagues and team members at Translucent You for the last ten years. I consider her a dear personal friend and inspiration. She is a model human being that truly walks the talk. Michelle is deeply committed to furthering and enhancing the quality of life of everyone she touches socially, not just in her practice. Every principle Michelle presents, every tool offered, I know she has tested. She wants to ensure it is legitimate, that it will strengthen and empower your body, mind, and spirit, your essence of wholeness.

Wellness is found in assisting people, in receiving their integral self and nurturing every aspect of that integral self for a happy, full, and human experience. Michelle knows that both the body and the heart must tick, must come together in collaboration for a human being to truly experience wellness in every part of their life. She is an expert at not only the mechanics of the human body, but the matrix of the human spirit. We separate them in our minds, yet they are not separate in reality. Unless we address both, we will not make strides to reach our optimal self.

Michelle is practical, responsible, and busy. She understands the constraints of time. Her approach to wellness is that the to-dos are naturally rewarding so that they don't feel like work or sacrifice. That mindset makes self-responsibility a pleasure, not a burden. The ideas she presents, if put into action, almost create a means of stretching time as we feel better and can get more out of each moment of our lives. However, Michelle makes it clear that, as much as she cares, there is no one out there that is more interested in our well-being than us. It starts and ends with us. She challenges us to flip the word responsibility and uncover its true meaning – the ability to respond. If we listen to our hearts, bodies, and spirits, and respond to our innate needs, we will build wellness. We forget that self-care is a positive quality. It is too often accepted that doing for others is better than caring for oneself. That's not accurate. Self-care should come first. It is a paradigm shift to take care of self and love that experience. Then there is an obligation to enhance the physical, mental, social, and spiritual well-being from the inside out, for self and then others.

There is a distinction between knowing about something or knowing information, and knowing from experience. Michelle's approach is seductive enough that you want to try it, yet practical enough that you will be able to do it.

And it works. I know because she restored me to health and wholeness. I have never felt better! She helped me transform my well-being even with my busy life; and I don't know anyone busier than me. Maybe you.

Health and wellness means wholeness and happiness. Anyone would come to this realization anyway. Michelle guides you to what you already intuitively know and helps you bring it forth in your life. I encourage you to read this book cover to cover. Then go back and read it in bite size chunks, really showing up to it, the concepts and the work, every day. In no time it will become the bedrock of your existence as it will lead you back to the wholeness you are intended to be.

Love and blessings,

Sonia Choquette

New York Times best-selling author, *The Answer Is Simple*
Speaker and Healer
Six Sensory Wisdom
www.soniachoquette.com

INTRODUCTION

Since the release of my first book, *Wellness on a Shoestring: Seven Habits for a Healthy Life*, in 2010 (second edition 2011), I have been blessed by the stories of positive wellness shifts in the lives of clients, friends, and strangers alike. *Wellness on a Shoestring* focuses on getting back to basics; taking the complexity out of being healthy by understanding the why and how of seven simple, cost effective, healthy habits that will fundamentally improve your mind-body-spirit well-being. I have shared the seven habits and supported thousands of people across the country in their wellness journey by speaking at conferences, companies, and churches as well as giving workshops and facilitating an 8-week program that accompanies the book (for more information visit www.DrMichelleRobin.com). It has been an honor.

In the last two years, I have heard many stories about seeking wellness that have led me to share a different perspective; hence this second book. Three key factors emerged: fully engaging a wellness lifestyle from the very core of who we are; understanding and maximizing energy in our physical bodies, our environments, and our mental space; and, enriching our lives through global connectivity, relationships, service, and gratitude. This book explains each of these concepts and what they can mean in your life as *real health changing factors* throughout your wellness journey.

I was inspired to write *Wellness on a Shoestring* partially as a response to clients seeking wellness but who were confused by the muddled, complicated noise of so-called solutions with which our society bombards us. What I was reminded of in the two years of promoting and teaching the book is that, as much as it reconnects readers to many of the basics of mind-body-spirit healthy habits and expands their understanding and practical application of those habits, it is not the first step of one's wellness journey. The heart comes before the basics. The heart, your true feelings and emotion, is at the core of decisions you make and changes to which you will commit. You can logically make decisions, yet the will of your heart will eventually overrule. Haven't you heard people say "her heart wasn't in it?" No matter how much you know about health and wellness, and to some degree no matter how much action you take, you will not make true progress in your journey if you don't address the heart of the matter.

The first factor, engaging a wellness lifestyle, starts with knowing your *why*. Why does it matter? Why will you do what you need to do to make a lasting change in your mind-body-spirit well-being? This *why* is why this time will be different, the first step. The next step of your wellness journey is setting intention. Having a clear vision of how you will act, approach life, feel, look and move, not just at the end – because there really isn't an end – but throughout the journey. The third step is planning your path. What are you going to do? The habits I talk about in *Wellness on a Shoestring* can be part of your path, starting with "Free Your Space" (Chapter 4 of *Wellness on a Shoestring*). The final step is to find your tribe. All of us need a support system of friends, family, health care providers, and others. Some of these people may not currently be in your life. I can tell you that without my tribe I am far less likely to get out of bed to work out and would probably have never dreamed of participating in a triathlon or biking across Iowa. These four elements of engaging a wellness lifestyle comprise the first health factor I will discuss.

The second factor addressed is *energy*. When new clients come to me, the two complaints I hear most often are back/neck pain – I am a Chiropractor after all – and a lack of energy. Pain and energy are not mutually exclusive. However, there are numerous reasons for low energy – some are physiological and others are not. In this section of the book I'll cover some of the physical sources of energy debits and credits such as adrenal fatigue and nutrition. I will also discuss the mental, emotional, spiritual, environmental and metaphysical elements of energy that have just as much impact as the physical. You will be surprised at the change in your overall health when you heighten your awareness of and manage the energy in your life in all its forms.

My story is a love story. Yes, if you read the introduction in my first book, you know that much of my childhood was challenging, like many of you. I had feelings of unworthiness. However, I was also blessed with the love of so many wonderful people in my community. It was through their love that I knew I could do anything I wanted. I was introduced to Chiropractic and what has become my passion – to inspire others to connect to their wellness. The last thirty years of being surrounded by wellness – learning, living and sharing it – has truly been a love story, steeped in gratitude, which has enriched my life and the lives of others. I get to pay it forward every day.

The third health changing factor is about enriching your life through community, relationships, gratitude and service. Realize that your health and well- being is bigger than you. That is not meant to put any pressure on you. It is just an acknowledgement that none of us, you or me, are isolated. We are all part of the greater whole. You've seen the news and statistics and heard the political debates swirling around the state of health and health care in the United States and the world. This is not something that can be solved by political legislation. It starts with each of us taking responsibility for our own health and understanding how we can impact our families, communities and society as a whole. Taking care of you is taking care of others. It is another version of "Think global. Act local." Knowing and seeing how improving your own well-being influences the world around you is a tremendously life-enriching experience. Next, focus on your relationships – romantic, family, friends, co-workers. Positive, mutually supportive relationships of all stripes enrich our day-to-day lives. People need people, to paraphrase Barbra Streisand in *Funny Girl*. Finally, enrich your life and those around you by being in gratitude and service of God and others. It is simple and true.

If you are thinking, "Umm… this health book isn't about diet, exercise and counting calories," you are right. It is not. Are a healthy, well balanced diet and active, exercise-infused lifestyle important parts of changing your health, especially if you need to lose weight? Yes. If you are looking for a life-altering shift in your health and your mind-body-spirit well-being, it is more than diet and exercise. You intuitively know this. But are you willing to take action, starting with your heart? I hope so. I hope that is why you are reading this book.

Throughout this book you and I will explore in more detail each of the health factors mentioned above, E factors, if you will – engage, energize, enrich. I will share with you what I have learned over the years, what I know to be true and what I have personally experienced or witnessed with my clients. Many of my clients have been generous, sharing their stories in these pages to exemplify their own E factors. I also will give you questions to ponder and practical action steps to take along your journey. You will find at the end of this book a list of resources for support and to continue learning.

Remember, this is a lifelong journey. You may set goals and milestones to achieve along the way, but there is no end point. It is because of this mindset that this book is not just for people who need to lose weight or have health challenges. It is also for people who would be considered fit and healthy. Just because you have developed the discipline to eat well and exercise doesn't mean you have fully embraced a mind-body-spirit wellness lifestyle, or that your life is energized and enriched in the ways we will discuss here. No matter where you are on your journey, this book is for you. Since this is a lifelong effort, you may think there is no rush. You can always start tomorrow. Aren't we often saying we'll start tomorrow? In fact, today is yesterday's tomorrow. Endless tomorrows will never come. And don't you want to start feeling better as soon as possible?

I encourage you to read this book, do the exercises and incorporate the action steps that work for you at your own pace. Step by step. Choice by choice. You will change your health and your life. Enjoy the journey!

Be well,

Michelle Robin, D.C.

Founder and Chief Wellness Officer
Your Wellness Connection, P.A.
Shawnee, Kansas

www.YourWellnessConnection.com
www.DrMichelleRobin.com

PART ONE

Engage A Wellness Lifestyle

Well-being is a lifelong journey that starts with your heart. Part One of this book begins with understanding what is at your core – the why and intention behind your journey – from your heart. Then I show you how to choose your path, and find a tribe of supporters and teachers to lead the way, walk with you and cheer from the sidelines. The four sections of Part One illustrate how you can engage a wellness lifestyle.

Chapter 1

Know Your Why

why [hwahy, wahy] *adverb, conjunction, noun, plural* whys, *interjection*

1. for what? for what reason, cause, or purpose?

2. a question concerning the cause or reason for which something is done, achieved, etc.

We are in the information age. A University of California, San Diego study in 2009 showed that the average American consumes 100,500 words in a typical day and processes 34 GB of information. [1] The sources of information are the usual suspects: radio, television, computer interaction, phone, books, magazines, people, and so on. Information is important. It can lead to knowledge. You are reading this book at the very least to gain knowledge or insight into health and wellness. One thing I know is that when it comes to improving your well-being, knowledge isn't enough (but don't stop reading). If it were we wouldn't have the health crisis, or many other issues, facing our society. Information alone does not lead to change. When it comes to health and wellness it starts with the heart, not the body's organ, but the intangible source of your *why*.

Let's take a little quiz. Which option in each pair in the following list is the healthier choice: Relaxation or stress? Calm or frustration? Exercise or couch potato? Clutter-free or messy space? Salad or French fries? Kids playing outside or channel surfing? Water or Diet Coke? Getting decent sleep or pulling all-nighters? Congratulations! I am rather certain you scored 100%! Yes, good health is more complicated than this quiz. However, the point is that you already know most of the basics and if you're a health information enthusiast you know quite a lot. So why aren't you putting it into practice? Why aren't you taking action? Why can't you seem to push past that one plateau? Why do you, as you may put it, keep sliding backwards? Why is your start date always next Monday and yet that intention never seems to stick? Why is it 2012 and you have made little or no progress towards the goals you may have set last year, three years ago, ten years ago?

I don't say any of this so that you will feel unsuccessful or start running the tapes in your head of blame, shame or excuses. I want you to understand that knowledge of what to do is not the starting point. You must know, or should I say feel, at your very core, deep in your heart the reason you want to be healthy and well – mind, body and spirit. Bring that heart-centered reason forward – from a feeling to a conscious knowing. This is your *why*. Know your *why*. Your own *why* is the reason this time that your efforts and results on your wellness journey will be different.

My history with my mom and determination to reach my potential are my *whys*. My birth was a surprise to my mom; she was not expecting twins. When she was in the delivery room on April 1 and had my brother, the doctor informed her there was another baby coming. My perception is that when the nurse named us my mom emotionally distanced herself, beginning my journey of pain and search for health. The message I received in my life with my heart was that I was a surprise and unwanted. Once again it is my perception that my mom has been in poor health the majority of my life. I have only heard her say she felt well three times, two of which were within the last year. If she said it more often than that I couldn't hear it. I was often told while growing up that she had been skinny and healthy until I was born; as if it were somehow my fault. Mom didn't take care of her health nor speak kindly to herself either.

I made peace with my mom in my heart many years ago. I love her, talk to her and visit her. Part of my *why,* why mind-body-spirit wellness is important to me, is that I want the opposite life experience I witnessed for my mom. I want health, movement, and positive, loving words and people surrounding me. I want joy. I have joy.

The second part of my *why* is the drive to fulfill my purpose and potential in life. I first experienced chiropractic care in high school after a sports injury. Mom had taken me to the hospital only to find that nothing was broken. The pain nonetheless didn't subside. Thank goodness she believed in chiropractic care and explored that approach to heal my injury. Through that experience and the connection I made with my chiropractor and his family, I knew this was my calling. My purpose has become more defined yet has broadened over the years. I know that I am meant to inspire people to live well. I do this through one-on-one client interactions, consulting to companies developing a wellness culture, and through speaking engagements and writing books and articles. This *why* is that I want to make the most of every day and have an impact on the well-being of as many individuals and communities as possible. Choosing wellness gives me the energy and health to fulfill this potential and lead by example.

> *Your time is limited; don't waste it living someone else's life. Don't be trapped by dogma, which is living the result of other people's thinking. Don't let the noise of other's opinion drown your own inner voice. And most important, have the courage to follow your heart and intuition, they somehow already know what you truly want to become. Everything else is secondary.*
>
> **- Steve Jobs**

What is your *why*? Why do you want to be holistically healthy – mind, body and spirit? What is the *why* at the core of your being that will make this time different? Is it that you want…

- to be able to enjoy your family more while they're young and be around as they get older?

- to play with your grandchildren?

- to take your healthy lifestyle to a new level, beyond diet and exercise?

- to be more active and have more energy?

- to be well without the use of drugs and medical intervention, saving money along the way?

- to live to your potential?

- to feel better, every day?

- to know you have control of your well-being?

- to truly love yourself?

Take note that if your *why* is something like 'to be more attractive for my partner,' or 'to never have to shop at a plus-size store again,' or 'so I can start dating', I challenge you to look deeper. Surface level reasons, especially those that are contingent on another person's actions, reactions or perceptions of you, will not be enough to drive your wellness journey forward for the long-term. If the initial *whys* that come forward are surface level, not only is there a truer, deeper why behind them, there are also other issues at play.

What is your *why*? Now, ask yourself how you will feel when you're far enough along the road to know you're different, when you have accomplished it, when it is your reality? Emotions motivate us.

EXERCISES

What do you want to stay the same in your life and what do you want to be different?

Think about all parts of your life – mind, body and spirit: your physical body, movement, activities, people, love, feelings, God/spirit, stress/calm, your environment/what surrounds you, how you eat, sleep, etc. Chart those ideas, actions, thoughts and feelings below.

What I Want to Stay the Same	What I Want to Be Different

My Why

_____

_____

_____

_____

Chapter 2

Set Your Intention

in ·ten ·tion [in-ten-sh*uh* n] *noun*

an act of determining mentally upon some action or result.

What Is Intention

The second part of engaging a wellness lifestyle is setting your intention. What do we mean by intention? Does it mean different things to different people? Is it something we experience and control individually or is it part of something bigger than us? Is intention something you think, feel, do, be or are part of? I say all of the above and possibly more.

Intentions are thoughts about what you want, expect to happen, do, or possibly feel and accomplish. We often make our intentions synonymous with our goals or vision for the future, i.e. I intend to go to graduate school; my intention is to clean out the garage this weekend; my intention is to be fit and active well into my 80s. People commonly use intention to indicate their desire or ideal situation, but don't necessarily always follow through. Their expression of intention, whether voiced or not, may only reside in thought and feeling while rarely resulting in action or whatever was originally desired. For others, intention is a mental and emotional commitment to action that will have a desired result. The primary difference is commitment to action; a *no matter what, I will make this happen or at least do everything I can to make progress* mindset. This person is the one who always keeps their word, not only to others, but to themselves. They may rarely commit to something, but when they do you know they are serious and will work at it until it comes to fruition. Still others see intention as their state of being. It is how they approach the world, proactively and responsively. Their intention is integrated in all aspects of their lives. You may see this in deeply spiritual people. Another example is someone that wholeheartedly lives for a cause, such as being "green." Their intention can be seen in how they shop locally for food, possibly garden, recycle, use reusable materials, conserve energy, and wear and use natural materials, etc.

All of the examples of intention I've described so far are all about you – your thoughts, feelings, actions, and way of being. I'd like you to consider intention as a community and the force that can create. Think of it as when a friend shares their dream with you and you in turn share the desire for them to reach that dream. We connect intentions when we 'hold space' for another's spoken need or aspiration. Community intention may manifest in a neighborhood's effort to make their streets and homes safe. While everyone involved may have independent intentions, they share a central intention of comfort and safety in community. There is a compounding effect of that awareness. Remember the potential impact of community intention when we talk about finding your tribe a little later in this book.

> *Let your intentions be good - embodied in good thoughts, cheerful words, and unselfish deeds - and the world will be to you a bright and happy place in which to work and play and serve.*
>
> **- Grenville Kleiser**

Now consider intention as Source, as Spirit. What if all of creation, literal and metaphysical, is intended to exist for the greater good? Dr. Wayne Dyer speaks of intention this way in his book, *The Power of Intention*. The intentions of Spirit are of the purest power and highest good. Just as there is a compounding effect of intentions when we join in community, imagine the amplification we can experience when our intentions are in alignment with our Source! It is like canoeing in a river. If your intentions, be they thoughts, feelings, actions or the whole of who you are being, are not for the highest good of self or others, you are paddling upstream. It is difficult. Life is hard. On the other hand, you may be focusing your intentions on the positive but are only partially embracing them or trying to do everything on your own. This would be like paddling in the river downstream but close to the bank. You're moving forward, but slower than others and running into obstacles and a jagged shoreline along the way. But what if you found your way to the center where the current is strongest and fastest? You would barely have to paddle at all. Yet every effort you made to stay with the central current, remaining steady and steering your canoe, would accelerate your momentum. You would be in the flow with power and speed beyond what you could do yourself. If you align, or surrender if you will, your intentions of thought, word, action and being to Spirit you will be in flow. Your goals, your mission, your vision, your intention of well-being will happen more smoothly and with an amplified grace you cannot achieve on your own. Intention exists on individual, communal and spiritual or universal levels.

Intention as Part of the Journey

You have likely heard the phrase 'It's the journey, not the destination.' The intentions you set can be both part of the journey and the destination. There is the place you are at today and the desired state of wellness. Your wellness potential lies in the gap. Your vision of self is part of your intention. The mindset and feelings with which you fulfill your wellness potential are part of your intention. The specific actions you take are your path, which we'll discuss in the next section.

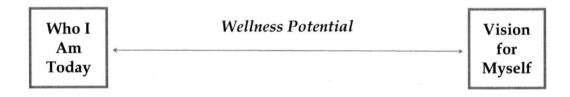

Intention is an important part of your journey to wellness. It creates the excitement and anticipation of what lies ahead both in the near-term and closer-than-you-think future. It will ground you in the present moment and remind you that the past is in the past. Intention also helps build your resistance to negative thinking and strengthen commitment to your path during difficult phases. The ability to focus on your intention will be a driving force throughout your journey. It will help you accomplish things you may not have thought you could do. While your *why* may be the purpose for your wellness journey, your intention(s) is the compass. It will keep you headed in the right direction.

Intention is woven into the scientific and spiritual law of attraction. The more you think, feel and live your intention throughout your journey, the more easily it will come to you. The tools, people, and resources necessary will show up as you need them. You will attract more of that which you choose to surround yourself. Use your intention as a guide throughout your journey.

> *What I know for sure is that your life is a multipart series of all your experiences - and each experience is created by your thoughts, intentions, and actions to teach you what you need to know. Your life is a journey of learning to love yourself first and then extending that love to others in every encounter.*
>
> **- Oprah Winfrey**

Set Your Intention

Setting your intention for your wellness journey is a process of creative visualization that may manifest itself as goals to be achieved, experiences to be had, or ways of being; it will likely be all of the above. I'm going to share a few questions you can answer to guide you through this process. Even if you think you know your intention this moment, I encourage you to take the time to go through the exercise below. If nothing else, it will confirm and clarify what you have already identified.

Earlier, I said your wellness potential lies in the gap between who you are today and the vision you have for yourself in the future. The first element of setting your intention is having a clear vision of your future. This is a multi-sensory vision – how you will feel emotionally, feel physically, look, and move. Your vision isn't really about an end point that is reached and then finished. Instead it is about a desired state of being that emerges throughout the journey. It is more than goal setting, but a vision of the whole experience of who you want to be and what you want to do. Then, consider how your intention is connected to community and the Universe/Spirit. Spend some time thinking about and responding to the questions below.

EXERCISES

Visioning

Get comfortable and quiet. Imagine your most ideal life scenario, a specific event, experience or general state of being. What's happening? What are you doing? What can you see, hear, smell, touch and taste? How do you feel physically? How do you feel in your body? What do you look like? How do you feel about yourself? Who is in your life? How are they in your life? Is there a Spirit connection in your life? How do you eat, sleep, or move? How do you practice self-care? What other thoughts and feelings do you have in the vision?

In the space below write a first person narrative ("I/we" statements) of your vision.

_____

_____

_____

_____

_____

_____

_____

_____

_____

_____

_____

_____

_____

_____

_____

_____

_____

_____

If you were to summarize your vision into one or two sentences, what would they be? What are the underlying themes of your vision written above? This is your intention.

My Intention (Think? Feel? Do? Be?)

_____

_____

_____

_____

_____

How is your intention connecting you to community and in alignment with Spirit?

_____

_____

_____

_____

_____

_____

Chapter 3

Plan Your Path

path [path, pahth] *noun*

1. a route, course, or track along which something moves.

2. a course of action, conduct, or procedure.

3. a continuous curve that connects two or more points.

You envisioned yourself in a state of wellness and set your intention in the previous section of this book. You know where you are going. Your intention is the compass that keeps you moving in the right direction. Now, how are you going to get there? The third element to engaging a wellness lifestyle is planning your path – the steps you will take on your journey to wellness.

Think about how you prepare for and get happily anxious when a big vacation is coming up. You're excited about what you'll experience along the way, yet realistic about how long each leg of the trip will take. You pack your suitcase and the car with everything you know you will need, plus extra this and that just in case. While you may not be able to predict every bend in the road, you can be clear from the outset, the main markers for which to watch and what turns to take. You may plan to stop for dinner in that town famous for everything Swedish or spontaneously stop to check out the world's biggest ball of twine. You listen to audio books or sing out of tune to your favorite songs. Even if you encounter a flat tire, road construction or a detour, eventually you get to your destination already having had an adventure. Your experience will be similar on the wellness journey you are about to begin, or begin anew. This is exciting! You are forging a new path that will lead you to a life of well-being beyond anything you've had before. There are a few things to keep in mind when planning and setting out on your wellness path.

Preparing for the Journey

As Stephen Covey said, "Begin with the end in mind."[1] Remember this journey is about wellness. Wellness is more than the absence of disease and ill health. It is a dynamic state of mind-body-spirit well-being in which you will progress toward a higher level of functioning resulting from optimal health and quality of life. The intention you set is your desired state of well-being – your goal – and this will serve as your compass. However, it is not a point on a map;

you are in uncharted territory. There is no decisive track or clear distance from point A to B. Yet you have the benefit of knowing the paths taken by others and having the tools to help along the way. Your journey to wellness is an exploration of who you are and who you want to become.

This journey is long, actually life-long. Most of my clients have complicated health and wellness issues. I often tell them to expect to take three years to reach just their initial wellness goals. At that time, new intentions may be set or finely tuned. There are also milestones of achievement along the way to encourage you and confirm your direction. As you set forth on your path, remember the words of the Taoist teacher, Lao Tzu, who said, "The journey of a thousand miles begins with a single step." Don't be discouraged by an anticipated lengthy duration of the journey. Be encouraged that, choice by choice and day by day, you are moving along the path toward your own personal vision of wellness.

Wellness is cumulative. It is like a bank account with credits, debits and compounding interest. Each choice, each action, each thought either adds to your mind-body-spirit well-being or subtracts from it. The next choice, action or thought either credits your wellness account or debits it. And the next. If we're talking about your actual bank account, the more you add to it the more capable you are of spending something for a treat or handling a major expense without going broke. The same is true for your health and wellness account. The more you build up your mental, emotional, spiritual, and physical well-being, the more you have to spend. You will have the energy to do everything you want, the capacity to love and be loved, a stronger faith, and the ability to heal quickly and resist illness. Wealth in wellness affords you the internal resources for both the joys and the difficulties in life. Positive actions and thoughts that credit your wellness account accumulate, and with compounding interest. Today, you may be able to only walk to the end of your street and back. But if you walked that short distance every day, by the end of the month you would likely be circling the block twice. When you break down your overall goals into manageable chunks, as you will in planning your path, you will feel the accumulation of health. As you begin to add more healthy choices while maintaining habits you've already created, it is as if you are gaining the compounding interest of health. So keep in mind how everything we think and do credits or debits our well-being. Take it day by day, choice by choice.

> *Nothing is impossible; the word itself says "I'm possible!"*
>
> **- Audrey Hepburn**

The easiest way to make progress with each choice, moving forward every day, is to be realistic about incorporating new habits into your life. Most likely what you've been doing and your current state of being have not led you to your desired state of wellness; that's why you're reading this book. Something has to change. Change can be difficult, especially when it involves altering long engrained habits, thought patterns, comforts, even traditions. Each of us responds to change differently. Be realistic about how you best cope with change when planning your path. It is common in our society to jump in with both feet and expect big results fast. We see all the possibilities, all the 'to dos' and options and we do them all at once and to an extreme. Unless you're in a crisis situation, being directed by your doctor to do something extreme right now, slow yourself down. Various studies have shown that it takes 21 to 30 days to change a habit. Small lasting changes that keep you on course are better than big brief changes that knock you off your path.

It is also easier to add in the good; in doing so, you eventually crowd out the bad. Let's say you have a diet soda addiction which is something you'd like to cut out in your wellness plan. Instead of cutting off or limiting the soda you consume in a day, commit to adding in X amount of water each day. If you're committed to the water, you will cut back on the soda – first out of necessity (after all there is only so much fluid one can drink in a day), and then because you will feel the benefits and prefer water over soda. When planning your path, initially identify those changes that are the best balance between (a) making a great impact on your health and well- being, and (b) doing something you can genuinely and consistently do, act, and think differently. Be honest with yourself on how you, yourself, best adopt change. Don't try to do it all at once. Take an 'add in the good' approach. You will get further faster when you make easier individual choices day by day.

Finally, in preparation for planning your path, understand that you don't have to know precisely how to reach your goals and live your intention when you set out on your journey. All you need to know is the next best step. It is okay to figure it out as you go without a clear, established plan in place. Let your intention be your guide. On the other hand, if you are the planning type and want to map it out in detail covering the next few months or years, that might work for you. Know that what you plan now may not be the direction you end up going; that is fine too. Your wellness journey is not a rigid project plan. It is a journey, which by its nature is somewhat unpredictable, and will curve, bend, pause, race and hit a stride. You just need to start. Then listen to your body and your spirit. Use your intention as your compass. You will change your approach or direction now and then as you are guided by the knowledge you gain and the feedback you get from body and spirit. That is okay, great in fact, because you're connected to your wellness and moving forward. You can't course correct if you aren't moving. So let's get moving!

Plan Your Path

Free Your Space

You are about to start on your path to mind-body-spirit wellness. You will shift your life, shake things up, add in a lot of good and crowd out the bad. You might need to clean house – literally and figuratively – in order to make room for the new you. I call this freeing your space. Freeing your space of clutter is a great place to start when planning your path. It gives you the opportunity to release what does not serve you, lighten up and make room for the new and positive or simply create openness.

Let me define space. I'm speaking of space as any area that you occupy or surrounds you physically or metaphysically. Spaces are your environments (i.e. house, car, and possessions), your physical body, and your mental, spiritual and emotional self. Clutter is anything that blocks you from living optimally in these spaces. As I shared in these excerpts from "Free Your Space" in *Wellness on a Shoestring*, "You may experience many different types of clutter during your life: There is spiritual clutter, which can keep you from being who you truly are. You may have mental or emotional clutter stemming from the beliefs of your parents which leaves you stuck in the past or worried about the future and unable to fully enjoy the present. You may also have clutter in your body, such as toxins stored in your liver or fat cells, or simply foods in your diet that don't work with your body chemistry. Any of these elements can make it harder for your body to function. One of the most powerful things you can do to support your own wellness is the regular elimination of what does not support or nurture you.

> *You is kind. You is smart. You is important.*
>
> **- Character, Aibileen Clark, in *The Help* by Kathryn Stockett**

"And then there is the clutter of things that people put between themselves and other people, and between themselves and new experiences. Do you touch your partner lovingly as you sleep, or do you always have a pet or pillow between you? Is there so much going on in your calendar that you have no white space, no downtime and no space for something new to come into your life?

"Clutter disconnects you from yourself, from your heart, and keeps you living a life in which you are not paying attention. You live looking in at all the mess, and you never have the energy to look out and around you, able to access what could bring you a better life. But don't despair: Wellness increases naturally and easily as you get rid of the clutter. And cleaning out your life doesn't have to happen all at once, in one huge cleansing session; it can and does happen bit by bit. Also, know that when you de-clutter your environment and your emotional self, you get rid of the noise that can keep you from being able to hear your inner wisdom or connect to a higher self or God. De-cluttering other parts of your life gives your mind and body, literally and figuratively, the space to be open, to have a dialogue with God, to connect with your spirit and receive the gifts of the Spirit."[2]

Freeing your space is an important part of your wellness journey. Much of it will happen naturally as you make wellness choices. You may choose to tackle specific clutter – environment, physical, spirit/emotional – as part of your planned path. Other clutter will have to be addressed along the journey as it becomes a significant obstacle to your progress. You'll know what, how and when to free your space when the time comes.

The Four Quadrants of Well-being

When I was studying chiropractic, I had the great fortune of being trained in acupuncture by Dr. Richard Yennie. His journey began as an eight year-old boy in the 1930's. Curious about Japanese, he took a bus across town to the Kansas City Public Library where he taught himself the language over time. As a young man, he found himself in Japan in 1949, where he served as a Japanese language interpreter at the Far Eastern Tribunal War Crimes Trials and as a Special Agent in the 441 Counterintelligence Corps after World War II. While in Japan, Yennie continued his Judo training at the Kodokan in Tokyo, where he sustained a serious low back injury during competition. After several weeks of conventional treatments in Yokosuka Naval Hospital were unsuccessful, Yennie's Judo teacher brought a master Japanese acupuncturist to his student. Yennie thought this old man in the long silk robes had to be nuts as he pulled out a box of tiny needles from his kimono sleeve. The acupuncturist asked where the pain was and then proceeded to stick needles in Yennie's knees. The back pain was gone. Mesmerized, Yennie inquired about this thing called acupuncture that had just relieved his pain. He learned there are 361 energy points in the body that when stimulated can reduce pain and restore function, thereby treating over 2,000 conditions. Instantly, this American interpreter, who had planned to return to the United States for law school, had a new course in life. Yennie studied Traditional Chinese Medicine (TCM), returned to the United States and became a doctor of chiropractic. He continues to practice chiropractic, acupuncture and TCM, as he has for over half a century now. Dr. Yennie is credited with being a leader in Alternative Medicine. He founded the Acupuncture Society of America and has taught acupuncture to over 60,000 chiropractors, physicians and health practitioners of many specialties over the years.

When I studied under Dr. Yennie, I learned the four principles of Oriental healing. The first is Tui na, which translates as "push pull." It is an ancient approach of physical manipulation similar to modern chiropractic methods addressing the structure of the body, including the spine. The second principle is nutrition and herbal therapy. There are over 800 herbs used in TCM healing. Acupuncture is the third principle. It treats by tapping into the body's electrical system improving its capacity to heal itself. The last principle is Qigong, a practice of healing and energy medicine that uses mind-body-spirit techniques to cleanse, strengthen and circulate life-energy. Dr. Yennie teaches that it is the balance of all four principles that provides optimal health. A practitioner should consider all four elements when assessing and treating a patient. Over the last twenty years, I have incorporated these principles into my practice as the four quadrants of well-being: mechanical, chemical, energetic and spiritual/psychological.

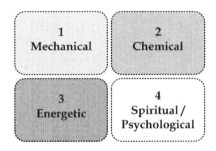

I practice client care in a holistic manner considering and addressing these four quadrants of health. As you plan your path for your wellness journey, bear in mind the four quadrants and ensure that you are caring for each. Earlier in this section, I wrote about the credits and debits in your whole body health account. As you increase your credits you help assure a healthy, positive balance. However too many debits will only lead to a negative bottom line and wellness bankruptcy. Think about how you may be currently crediting or bankrupting that part of your well-being, as we explore each quadrant.

1　　The Mechanical quadrant includes the needs of the physical or structural body: bone, muscles, ligaments, tendons and nervous system. Movement is core to the well-being of the mechanical quadrant to build strength and flexibility. My focus as a chiropractor is caring for the nervous system. The nervous system is the information superhighway between your brain and every cell, tissue, muscle, hormone, organ, etc., that controls every function of our bodies – absolutely everything. Keeping your nervous system in good working order is critical to optimal whole body health. Chiropractic removes nerve interference. Your medical doctor will not typically check your nervous system.

Our bodies are phenomenal. They are constantly self-healing and renewing. We have a new intestinal lining every five days. Every eleven days, our respiratory lining is replenished. Every eleven months, we have a new cell structure. Every part of our bodies refreshes and regenerates on its own cycle so that we have an entirely new body every seven years. However, we are rather harsh toward our physical bodies. We push them to the limit and often see pain, soreness and stiffness as battle scars about which we brag or consider proof that we gave our all. Yes, pain, soreness and stiffness, if temporary as an immediate response to working hard, playing sports, exercising and going that extra mile, are acceptable. However, it is not normal for the body to be in pain for extended periods. Pain, no matter how slight, is distracting to you consciously, and is harmful to your whole being working optimally, either consciously or sub-consciously. Pain is your body's last resort to get your attention! By the time you're feeling pain and discomfort, you likely have had an issue for quite a while. Dr. Roger Sperry, noted Nobel Prize winner in brain research says, *"The more mechanically distorted a person is, the less energy for thinking, metabolism and healing."* Your physical body will do amazing things for you. Take care of it.

Mechanical Quadrant	
Credits	**Debits**
• Good sleep posture	• Carrying heavy bags on one shoulder
• Regular health checkups	• Sitting too long in one position
• Chiropractic care	• Improper lifting of heavy objects
• Massage	• Talking on the phone without a headset
• Relaxation techniques	• Sleeping on your stomach
• Good ergonomics while sitting at your desk and in the car	• Sitting on your billfold
• Get movin'!	• Sleeping on a bad bed
• Your proper body weight (gaining lightness vs. losing weight)	• Hunched shoulders/poor posture

2   The Chemical quadrant focuses on the body's chemistry and efforts to stay in a state of homeostasis (balance). The body's chemistry is impacted by what enters the body and what is released. You are what you consume: food choices, beverages, supplements, medication, drugs (including nicotine). Nutrients from food are the top source for your body to be chemically balanced. Shop the perimeter of the grocery store – usually fresh and frozen sections – and eat whole foods. Processed foods are nutritionally depleted and loaded with unnecessary and unbeneficial chemical compounds. They are frequently heavy with Omega 6 fatty acids leading to excessive inflammation in the body. Your body chemistry is impacted by the content of the products you use on your skin in the shower, in your make-up, skin care, and sunscreen. Your body also absorbs toxins in the air, on the surfaces around you via cleaning products, and in containers that leach into food and beverages. I know it can seem

overwhelming, but every effort you make to consume 'clean' makes a difference.

As much as chemistry is affected by what is consumed, it is also altered by what is released. Our body is masterful with detoxifying systems, but those systems need to be adequately supported in order to work. There are many reasons for being adequately hydrated (see Chapter 7 of *Wellness on a Shoestring*); flushing out toxins via urine is one. If you have heard me talk or have met me you likely know how much I love to talk about pooping! Regular pooping is critical to your health as it removes waste products. Breathing isn't just about getting oxygen. It is also a detoxifying process that releases carbon dioxide and other unnecessary chemicals. Deep breathing releases toxic chemicals and stuck emotions out of the body and triggers the internal release of calming hormones that support the body (see Chapter 2 of *Wellness on a Shoestring*). Then there is sweat. The body loves to sweat as another process to remove waste. Get moving and get sweaty!

How we live and rest affects our chemistry as well. Stress and a lack of sleep shift our chemical balance. We will talk a little more about that in Part 2: Energize. Our bodies are brilliant chemists. Our job is to provide quality sources (i.e. nutritious food, water and supplementation) and do our best to avoid and remove toxins.

Chemical Quadrant	
Credits	**Debits**
• Adequate hydration – drink half your body weight in ounces daily	• Smoking
• Healthy breakfast daily	• Eating right before bedtime
• Good fiber, i.e., fruits, veggies	• Sugars and sodas
• Quality multi-vitamin	• Processed foods (Inflammatory foods)
• Whole, nutritious foods, especially veggies	• Excessive caffeine
• Alkaline diet	• Excessive alcohol
• Vitamin D	• Excessive/ongoing prescription drugs
• Chewing your food	• Not getting adequate sleep
• Omega 3 - plant based or fish oil	• Skipping meals

3   The Energetic quadrant centers on the subtle life-energy that courses through our body, our vital force. It is chi or qi to the Chinese, prana to Hindus. Sigmund Freud referred to it as libido. Many consider this Universal energy. It is physics and metaphysics. Everything is energy at the subatomic level that creates all matter. Everything has energy. We feel it when we meet people or walk in a room and 'get a vibe.' The trillions of cells in our bodies vibrate with a specific frequency of energy. Our internal energy interacts with external environments and energy sources. We give and receive energy. When that energy interaction and transfer is healthy, it is smooth and harmonious. We are healthy and balanced. We can feel it. When we are of ill health or low energy – mind, body, spirit – it is really an imbalance of energy between our internal and external environments. I wrote earlier in this section, there is a direct connection between energy and freeing your space.

There is an Alternative Medicine specialty called Energy Medicine. It uses energy fields such as electrical, magnetic, sonic, acoustic, microwave and infrared, in therapy. Practitioners use these therapies to screen for or treat health conditions by detecting and correcting imbalances in the body's energy fields. Nobel Prize winner, Albert Szent-Gyorgyi, said, "In every culture and every medical tradition before ours, healing was accomplished by moving energy." As you plan your path, include changes that will shift your energy. Raise your awareness of your energy and the energy around you throughout the journey. It will surprise you.

Energetic Quadrant	
Credits	**Debits**
• Acupuncture	• Television in the bedroom
• Safe and positive living conditions	• Cluttered, unorganized living spaces
• Reiki	• Lack of alone time
• Slow, deep breathing	• Loud noise
• Singing, smiling, laughing, and dancing	• Energy drains
• Good friendships	• Over-committed calendar
• Energy work	• Saying yes when you really want to say no
• Playing in the earth	
• Hot shower or bath before bed	

[4] The Spiritual / Psychological quadrant is the awareness that pain or dysfunction in the body can be associated with spiritual and emotional blocks. Some would consider this psychosomatic practice – the undeniable yet not fully understood connection between the physiology of the body and the psychology of the mind. This quadrant is beyond psychology however. There is a spiritual, soul-centered component to our being that also has an undeniable yet not fully understood connection to our bodies.

Your physical well-being is integrated with your mental, emotional and spiritual well-being. Stress is the most evident example. You experience stress mentally, emotionally, physically and even spiritually. It can initiate in any of those elements of our being yet impact the others. Dr. Hans Selye, a pioneering endocrinologist and expert on stress tells us, *"Every stress leaves an indelible scar and the organism pays for its survival after a stressful situation by becoming a little older."* We'll talk more about stress in Part 2: Energize when we discuss adrenal fatigue. It is also true that people who are happy, express gratitude and connect to something bigger than them – be that community, God, the Universe – are often healthier. You will read more about this in Part 3: Enrich. The lesson of this quadrant is that the spiritual and psychological aspects of your being are factors of your overall wellness. Include time and effort to address this quadrant as you plan your path.

Spiritual / Psychological Quadrant	
Credits	**Debits**
• Self love	• Lack of personal responsibility
• Positive mental attitude	• Inability to forgive – yourself and others
• Balance of work and play	• Selfishness / Selflessness
• Counseling / Coaching	• Lack of personal joy
• Meditation with a higher power	• Negative outlook on life
• Healthy touch	• Negative self-talk
• Gratitude	• Gossip

The four quadrants are interdependent. Anything we do will impact more than one quadrant if not all four in some way. Let's take sleep and low back pain as examples.

Sleep

1 Mechanical: Sleep enhances proper nerve function; or poor sleep posture can negatively impact nerve function.

2 Chemical: Sleep strengthens the immune system, and provides the appropriate increase and decrease of hormones such as melatonin and cortisol; a lack of sleep accelerates aging as it negatively impacts natural antioxidants like melatonin.

3 Energetic: Sleep allows for restoration and rejuvenation of the physical and metaphysical body, and conservation of energy stores in cells.

4 Spiritual/psychological: Sleep elevates mood, and recharges brain and cognitive function.

Low Back Pain

1. Mechanical: Some sources of low back pain can be bad shoes, sitting too long, tight muscles, spinal misalignment or a bad mattress to name a few.

2. Chemical: Low back pain may be a result of dehydration, constipation and/or adrenal fatigue.

3. Energetic: Pain in the lower back could indicate a lack of intimacy, or emotions such as fear or feeling frozen.

4. Spiritual/psychological: Feeling a lack of support, anger or an inability to manifest intentions and desires can present as low back pain.

Can you see the crossover and interdependence of the mechanical, chemical, energetic and spiritual/psychological elements of wellness?

I know you're ready to plan your path. I've shared a lot to ponder. Take it all in. Filter my suggestions for what is in alignment with your own intention and mind-body-spirit needs at this point in your journey. Remember: this is a marathon, not a sprint. In addition to the short lists of credits and debits shown with the description of each quadrant above, I've listed on the following pages the Seven Habits and other health changing wellness habits. Incorporating a few of these changes as part of your path will improve your well-being. Everyone is at a different place in their wellness journey. Therefore, some of the items listed cover a range of complexity, fitness levels, etc. As new habits become true for you, refer back to this list for new ideas to add even more and healthier habits to your life that can take you to the next level of mind-body-spirit wellness.

Seven Habits from Wellness on a Shoestring

1. Rest, Reflect, Rejuvenate –Sleep position, quantity of sleep, as well as rejuvenating activities and gratitude.

2. Breathe Deeply – Proper breathing affects the function of all bodily systems; meditation positively impacts mind-body-spirit.

3. Move Your Body – Movement enhances concentration, releases toxins, and maintains and increases range of motion.

4. Free Your Space –Removing physical, environmental and emotional clutter lightens your mind, body, and spirit.

5. Go for the Greens – Greens powerfully support your digestive system and cell functionality.

6. Eat from the Sea – Enjoy the Sun – Omega 3 and Vitamin D can boost energy and alleviate many pains and ills.

7. Drink to your Health –Adequate hydration with pure water is critical for functionality, removal of toxins, and refreshment of mind, body, and spirit.

Four Quadrant Wellness Habits

1   Mechanical

- Use a towel roll for stretching 5-10 minutes / day for flexibility
- Improve sleep posture:
  - Get a proper pillow that supports your neck in a neutral position
  - Sleep on your side with a pillow between your knees to support hips and lower back
  - Sleep on your back with a pillow under your knees to support lower back
  - No stomach sleeping or arms above the head
- Maintain proper posture while lifting
- Do not sit on your wallet
- Use a cold pack or moist heat pack as needed to sooth muscles and recuperate
- Take 3 deep breaths upon waking
- Do stretching exercises
- Get outside — walk, run, bike, hike

- Wear a pedometer and move 8,000 – 10,000 steps / day
- Get cardio exercise weekly at an adequate heart rate
- Get a massage
- Evaluate the ergonomics of your desk and / or car
- Replace running shoes frequently to avoid trauma to hips, knees and ankles
- Use a headset while talking on the phone
- Do nasal cleansing for sinus relief
- Do a 6 count breath in — hold — then release. Do 5x before bed
- Get spinal adjustments
- Do weight training
- Practice daily spinal hygiene
- Brush your teeth multiple times a day
- Floss daily
- Practice yoga

2 Chemical

- 2-5 pieces of fruit for breakfast along with protein
- 75% of food consumed is vegetables
- Drink half your body weight in ounces of water per day
- Drink hot water with lemon to make your body more alkaline
- Decrease caffeine intake to 2-3x / week maximum or eliminate all together
- Limit or eliminate smoking
- Limit or eliminate alcohol consumption
- Enjoy green smoothies for breakfast
- Take a quality multi-vitamin daily
- Take 1-2 digestive enzymes with each meal
- Take a probiotic
- Decrease refined foods, saturated fats, hydrogenated oils and high fructose corn syrup
- Shop the perimeter of the grocery store
- Keep refined sugar to a minimum
- Consume whole, nutritious foods
- Do not eat within 2 hours prior to going to bed
- Start juicing vegetables
- Do a 3 day detox monthly and a 10 day detox in the Spring and Fall
- Continue current supplements
- Take fish oil
- Take a vitamin D3 supplement
- Know your lab results
- Stay hydrated
- Eat organic as much as possible

3 Energetic

- Avoid watching television immediately prior to going to bed
- Take off jewelry prior to bed
- Take 5 deep breaths upon waking, before bed and in stressful situations
- Read a magazine you have never read before
- Read aloud with your partner; alternate who reads and who listens
- Read *The Energy Bus: 10 Rules to Fuel Your Life, Work and Team with Positive Energy*, by Jon Gordon
- Read *Healthy Sleep Habits, Happy Child*, by Marc Weissbluth
- Cover the television in your bedroom when going to bed, or remove the TV altogether
- Take a hot shower or bath before bed and visualize letting go
- Grow a garden
- Sleep 8 hours each night
- Consider Feng Shui for your house
- Rearrange familiar things in your office or on your desk
- Consider meditation
- Spend 30 minutes / day in quiet, alone time
- Create a regular sleep routine
- Experience reike
- Get a Lomi Lomi massage
- Get cranial sacral treatments
- Get acupuncture treatments

4 <u>Spiritual / Psychological</u>

- Work on your vision - what do you want your life to look like:
  - Health
  - Career
  - Family
  - Financial
  - Relationship
  - Spiritual
  - Other areas…
- Consider counseling or coaching services
- Don't watch the news before bed
- Read *The Negative Love Syndrome* and the *Quandrinity Model* (Hoffman Institute)
- Write daily 5-10 things for which you are grateful, shift thinking to positive frequencies
- Consider daily journaling
- Focus on the present moment
- Practice meditation
- Volunteer for something you believe in
- Spend time with people who fill you with joy

- Play the "I love…/ I am grateful for…" game
- State an affirmation each morning and throughout the day. For example:
  - My body is vibrantly healthy.
  - I am healthy and fulfilled. My life is flowing perfectly.
  - I feel safe and secure in the world. All my needs are being met.
  - I have a deep reserve of energy within me that nourishes my essence and creativity.
  - I handle my life issues in a balanced and self-confident manner.
  - Love flows through me. I give and receive love and caring in all of my relationships.
  - I communicate my needs freely and openly. I enjoy expressing myself.
  - I make time every day to relax and enjoy myself.

EXERCISES

Revisit Your Why and Intention

Go back to page 17 and revisit your *why* and page 26 for your *intention*. Rewrite them in the spaces provided below for easy reference. Your why and intention are your inspiration and guides as you plan your path.

My Why

_____

_____

_____

My Intention

_____

_____

_____

Free Your Space

For each area list ways you can free your space.

Area	I will free my space by...
Calendar	(e.g., leaving my calendar open after 8pm during the work week.)
Repairs, Mending and Maintenance	(e.g., sewing the button on my black pants; replacing the broken brick on the patio.)
Declutter	(e.g., purging and organizing the papers piled on my desk; cleaning out the refrigerator and freezer.)

Doubts and Negative Self Talk	(e.g., being aware of and limiting my use of *always* and *never*.)
People and Situations	(e.g., telling Annie I can't talk to her every night.)
Toxic Habits and Products	(e.g., quitting smoking; replacing cleaning products with earth friendly products.)

My 4 Quadrants

Note in each quadrant box actions you will take and changes you will make along your wellness path. You can list items you will do now or down the road. If an item impacts more than one quadrant list it in multiple spaces. This will help you identify some of the changes that may have the biggest impact on your well-being. You can reference the lists of suggestions on pages 45-48, the Seven Habits from *Wellness on a Shoestring* and the Free Your Space exercise on the previous pages for ideas.

Mechanical	Chemical

Energetic	Spiritual / Psychological

Prioritizing

1. Circle the items you listed in more than one quadrant.

2. Looking at all the items (not just the circled ones), put an X or asterisk (*) by those items that feel the most doable…those to which you feel you can commit to changing right now or in the near future.

3. Of the items you marked, mark a second time (with a different symbol) those you think would make the biggest impact on your well-being (mind, body, spirit).

4. In the **My Path** table that follows…

   a. List any items that are circled and have two marks.

   b. List any items that have two marks.

   c. List any items that were marked for doable only.

Does everything left in the quadrant boxes either seem: 1) to have little impact or 2) not doable? Either reevaluate your choice for not marking those items or leave them to be reconsidered at a later date.

My Path

Following the prioritization outlined above, write below the steps for your path following the headings for each column.

1. I Am Going to… describe the health and wellness change you are going to make.

2. Because… describe why you are making this change. What do you expect to experience?

3. Beginning… Is this something you can start right now or later at some point? Keep in mind that you want to limit the number of changes you make at once.

4. Quadrants… Mark (x) which quadrants you're addressing for each action. Note which quadrants, if any, have few or no marks. Is this because you feel balanced in that quadrant or have you overlooked it? Does this change your list?

5. Resources... Identify any resources you may need, i.e. new walking shoes, food processor, etc.

6. Now choose three (3) changes (*I Am Going to...* items) from the prioritized list and take the first step on your path!

Resources	Impacted Quadrants				Beginning	Because... *Why*	I Am Going to... *What, When, How, Where*
	Energetic	Spiritual / Psychological	Chemical	Mechanical			

What's Next

Revisit the My Path plan frequently to recommit to the changes you've chosen to make, to be reminded of the big picture, or to consider the next steps on your path. Now and then throughout your wellness journey, on a time frame that works best for you, rework all the exercises in this section. You will be in a different place along your path. That will change your perspective as you work through the exercises. Your answers to the questions and the new habit choices you make for the next leg of your journey will be different.

Chapter 4

Find Your Tribe

tribe [trahyb] *noun*

any aggregate of people united by ties of descent from a common ancestor, community of customs and traditions, adherence to the same leaders, etc.

Spending time taking care of yourself, walking your own path, does not mean you have to do it alone. In fact, it is better if you have a tribe. Typically when we think of tribe we picture native or aboriginal peoples, focusing primarily on the ancestral connection. We may assume that definition translates to our tribe being our family and friends. Yes, and beyond. Author Seth Godin tells us that a tribe is simply "a group of people connected to one another, connected to a leader and connected to an idea." He goes on to say that "A group needs only two things to be a tribe: a shared interest and a way to communicate."[1]

Beyond your family, you are certainly part of a number of tribes: alumni group, book club, PTA, golf buddies, neighborhood, choir, country club, church, Mac (vs. PC people), iPhone (vs. Android people), Comic-con, political party, networking groups, etc. The internet creates a myriad of new ways to form tribes. Think about your social media habits: how you group friends on Facebook, the circles you form within Google+, who you follow on Twitter, blogs you follow, or the groups you join on LinkedIn. In all of these examples you have a shared interest or intention for coming together, being in alignment with one another.

I'm Fine On My Own

Why do we form tribes and why do we do it the way we do? There are entire fields of study in social, behavioral, natural and complexity sciences to answer those questions. In 1943, Abraham Maslow published an article, "A Theory of Human Motivation," in *Psychological Review*, which he later expanded upon in books and detailed what he deemed a hierarchy of needs. Let's consider Maslow's Hierarchy of Needs[2] for insight strictly from the perspective of your wellness tribe. Maslow's theory surmised that humans had five primary needs: physiological, safety, love and belonging, esteem, and self-actualization. He believed that, in order for one to move towards self-actualization, the other needs must be met and in the order listed.

Hierarchy Level *Lowest to Highest*	Corresponding Needs
Physiological	Having enough food and water, sex for reproduction, breathing, sleep, homeostasis, release of toxins/excretion
Safety	Security of body, resources, health, property/shelter, family
Love and Belonging	Family, sexual intimacy, friendship, connectedness
Esteem	Confidence, achievement, self-esteem, respect of and from others
Self-Actualization	Problem solving, innovation, creativity, spontaneity, morality, free of prejudice, acceptance of fact

You can imagine how beneficial it was to be part of a tribe thousands of years ago, even hundreds of years ago. A tribe made it easier to have enough food, secure shelter, and protection from wild animals and other tribes. The tribe was family, intimacy and community. Depending on the tribe and point in history, there may have been a hierarchy in leadership or status to achieve. The evolution of civilization demonstrates levels of self-actualization reached. Fast forward centuries and tribes are the communities we are either born into or choose. While the primary reason for being part of a tribe may no longer be survival, community is still a critical part of reaching self-actualization. That is why a tribe which echoes your quest for wellness is important.

Physiologically, your wellness tribe may support you by: teaching you about nutrition, preparing and eating healthier foods, encouraging you to drink more water, guiding you through a detox, helping you sleep better, and learning to meditate and breathe more deeply. In terms of safety, your tribe may support you by: further care of your health, teaching you proper techniques when you begin new exercises and sports, being your spotter when rock climbing, or as your physical therapist helping you rebuild flexibility.

A wellness tribe will provide the support, love and belonging that help along your journey. Your own wellness tribe connects you to others of like-mind and ambition, and will support development of your habits. Dan Buettner traveled the world researching communities (tribes) where people were living the longest and healthiest lives or Blue Zones as he calls them. The only Blue Zone in the United States is a Seventh Day Adventist community in Loma Linda, California. There are many ways of living that contribute to the long lives of Adventists, one of which is, as Buettner states in his book, *Blue Zones: Lessons for Living from the People Who've Lived the Longest*, "Adventists tend to spend lots of time with other Adventists. They find well-being by sharing values and supporting each other's habits."[3] They have many community members living past 100, so they must be doing something right. I can tell you that without my tribe sharing my values and habits, I am far less likely to get out of bed to workout and would probably have never dreamed of participating in a triathlon or biking across Iowa.

What could be better for your esteem than your own fan club? Those in your tribe will cheer you on so loudly they'll drown out any self-doubt still chanting in your head. It is often difficult for us to acknowledge how much we've achieved when all we can see is how far we have to go. Your tribe will see and praise your accomplishments even when you can't. As it states in Proverbs 27:2, "Let another praise you, and not your own mouth; a stranger, and not your own lips." That is not to say self-acknowledgment isn't wonderful; it is. But positive recognition from others further feeds our motivation. You know what it is like if you ever dieted and felt the weight was coming off at the speed of a slug and not noticeable, until you run into someone you hadn't seen for months. They noticed the change right away. Hearing it from them brightened your day.

Finally, your tribe will support the highest needs of self-actualization. The new level of physical, mental and emotional confidence you will gain along your path will inspire you to be bold. Your tribe will be a source of that inspiration and spontaneity as well as be by your side as you take on new adventures. As you get further along your wellness journey, you will inevitably gain clarity about many things in your life, such as relationships with others, with your health, in your heart and even in your relationship with God. You'll have a clearer understanding of the past, a more grounded reality check on the present and an unobstructed view of the future. Your wellness tribe will be part of that clarity as the fog lifts and the light enters.

Hopefully you can see how your tribe may weave in and out of your wellness journey and provide for your needs along the way. Although descriptive, my explanation above is not the only way a tribe will support you. It is just a snapshot. Your tribe, like you, like your why, intention and path, will be unique and tailored to your needs and desires. It will also change throughout the journey. Who and what you need now may be different from three months or three years from now. That's okay. That's life.

Finding Your Wellness Tribe

Your wellness tribe is anyone, any community, online or in-person, that actively supports or adds to your wellness journey. Your tribe is connected by the shared interests that relate back to your intention and path. That is not to say that everyone in your tribe must know your intention or the details of your path, nor even know you personally. It is a customized mishmash of people that simply share an interest related to your wellness journey, about which you communicate and engage. As an example, your tribe may include your primary care physician who is aware of all things medical; and it may also include the running club you joined whose members just share their love of running.

When you think about the composition of your tribe, consider the path you identified in the last chapter. Build your tribe based on the elements of your path, what you recognized as needs and goals for each of the four quadrants as well as freeing your space. You don't have to know who or how your tribe will come together to start moving on your path. It isn't like putting together a baseball team with every position filled before the game can start. While some of the members of your tribe will know each other, most won't. If part of your tribe is an online community, you may not even know them, as odd as that sounds. Some of your tribe will be your oldest and dearest friends, family and care providers. Some may not currently be in your life at all. If you go back to the beginning of this chapter, Godin tells us that all you really need is a shared interest (you and/or your goals), a leader (you as the center) and a way to communicate. Where to start? Let me share an example.

My friend Valerie Thomas is in her late thirties. She is morbidly obese with back and knee problems along with a number of other health issues, including adrenal fatigue and hormone imbalance. She hates to exercise. Valerie has already taken a number of health and nutrition classes, but isn't great about compliance with her own goals. She is taking a new approach starting with her why, intention and path. I asked her to outline her tribe as she sets out on this new leg of her journey. She listed:

- Health Care Providers: a concierge medical doctor, me as her chiropractor

- Physical Activity/Exercise: a friend that is a triathlete and coaching her for the WIN for KC mini-triathlon; several friends that are also training for the mini-tri; her local community center gym; a few friends that will go for walks now and then

- Spiritual: becoming more involved with her Church, signed up for an hour of adoration each week

- Mental/Emotional: starting a blog to share her journey (www.myrightthigh.com); she updates friends and that cheer her on via email; she occasionally visits with a counselor; several blogs and Facebook pages she follows for inspiration and information on health and well-being

- Food and Nutrition: friends that will go to healthier places when eating out; friends that will cook healthy meals together

Valerie's tribe is an example of what will work for her at this stage of her journey. It is time for you to determine who and what will work for you. Remember all the ways a tribe will benefit your mind-body-spirit wellness along your path. It is a kaleidoscope of love, support, expertise, companionship and a personal fan club. Enjoy!

EXERCISES

Your Wheel of Support

You are the hub of your wellness tribe, a wheel of support. Who surrounds you? Go back to pages 49 and 55 to review your *why, intention* and *path*. The direction and goals you've laid out will help you determine who or what would be beneficial as part of your wellness tribe.

In the figure:

1. Identify the different types of members or communities you need. I've started it for you. The number of segments/spokes does not matter, so tailor it to your needs.

2. List – on the lines connecting YOU to each labeled and unlabeled spoke, list the individual people or groups you either have currently or want to seek out as part of your tribe. Remember, you get to choose who is in your wellness tribe. Just because someone is family or a longtime friend does not mean you have to consider them part of this tribe. It will also change over time.

Wheel of Support

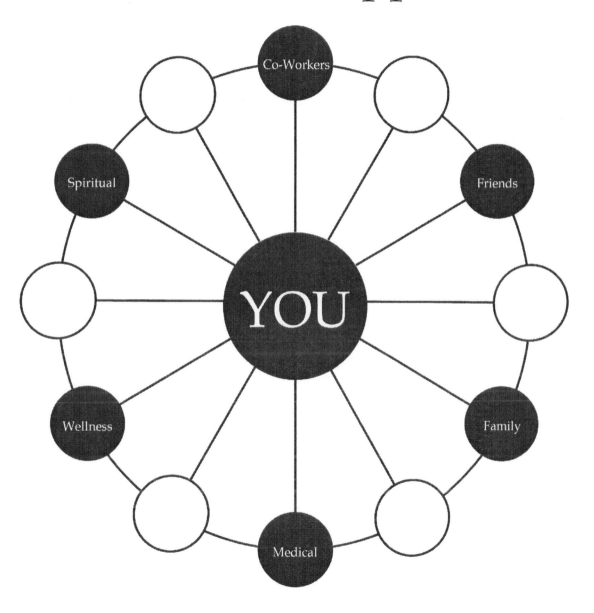

Personal Stories

Amy Gross

Amy Gross is in her late forties. She was about 100 pounds overweight, with stiffness, back and joint pain. She has been a client for over twelve years. The last several years I'd asked her if she were ready to work on the rest of herself, beyond her alignment and mechanical health. She was not. Then last year Amy came to me and said she was ready. She realized how deeply unhappy she was and wanted to truly change her mind-body-spirit well-being. She wanted to be happy.

I invited Amy to a screening of "May I Be Frank" where the star and film director, my friends, Frank Ferrante and Gregg Marks, would be for commentary and questions. It is a powerful documentary film about the holistic transformation of Frank himself. It is a testament to the fact that for many, or dare I say all of us, losing weight and becoming well is not about diet and exercise alone; it starts with the heart. Amy came to the screening. Before we began we passed out little Sweet Pea cards with positive sayings. The one Amy received said, "Expect to fall in love every day." It really touched her as she realized how much she didn't love herself. She cried throughout the film and on the way home. Amy set her intentions from that point forward to fall in love with herself every day.

The next time I saw Amy she told me about her experience seeing the film. This time when I asked if she were ready she said 'yes.' In her career, Amy is an event planner and caterer. She is on her feet cooking, organizing, making things happen eight, ten, twelve, up to seventeen hours a day. It is a stressful life that ebbs and flows with seasons of celebration. I asked Amy what the next couple months looked like and the stress level she was expecting. It was going to be a crazy busy quarter. I told her to wait. She was about to embark on a rather significant shift, something for which she would want time and focus. She should expect it to be a three-year process to reach her goals, but also a lifelong journey. We set a start date. I saw Amy several times before that. She was anxious to get going. Amy had tried all the fad diets and national weight-loss franchises over the years. They didn't stick. She told me she knew this time would be different because her reasons and intentions were different. Her reason, her *why*, was to be happy. Her intention, her goal, was to fall in love with herself every day. And for the first time she felt that someone outside of her immediate family truly cared about her well-being and was willing to invest time and effort to support her. She had a tribe.

Our start day arrived. Amy met with our YWC wellness coach, Shelly Murray, HHC, AADP, and Crystal Jenkins, LCPC, one of our counselors, and me. The first step was a four-week detox. Amy shared that after making it through the discipline of the detox she knew she had the fortitude to make lasting changes. Clearly, as a caterer, Amy has an extensive knowledge of food as a creative and delicious force. However, Amy met with Shelly for integrative nutrition coaching to understand and see food differently. Now she looks at her food choices for how they make her feel and fuel her body, when she used to eat for no reason at all or for every reason in the book. Amy has spent time with Crystal and come to the acceptance that she is enough and worthy of happiness and health, freeing her mind and heart space of beliefs that don't serve her. We have been fortunate enough to be part of Amy's tribe and journey.

Amy continues on her journey. After a few short months she tremendously improved her energy level, decreased her swelling and joint pain, and lost nearly 40 pounds. She sees and chooses food differently, now gluten, dairy and sugar-free. She approaches her journey choice by choice, day by day. Every day she reads her Sweet Pea card as a reminder to fall in love, with herself, every day…and she has.

Amy's …

Why: Happiness and love of self.

Intention: Fall in love with myself every day.

Path: Nutritional coaching; gluten, dairy, and sugar free diet; counseling to realize I am enough and can be happy now versus later; learning to love myself.

Tribe: Friends, sister, my YWC family.

Karen Birdsall

All was well in Karen Birdsall's life, or so it seemed. Sure, she had stress at work, but doesn't everyone? She was rather healthy and made an effort to eat well with whole, balanced nutrition. Emotionally, that balance did not exist. Her world was always a pass/fail, black/white, all/nothing radical pendulum swing of control and perfectionism. One day, seemingly out of the clear blue sky, Karen collapsed on the floor. She was spinning, which induced nausea and vomiting. Everything around her was in rotation, whirling by like helicopter blades. She had an onset of severe vertigo. Karen literally crawled back in bed and didn't leave her horizontal haven for a week.

Continuing to experience vertigo after a week, Karen started seeing doctors. She made the rounds going to an Ear, Nose and Throat specialist, an audiologist, the ER, and a general practitioner. She even had an MRI to confirm there weren't any tumors or clogged arteries causing the imbalance. There were no answers found. She was given pharmaceutical drugs to relieve the symptoms of vertigo and nausea, as well as Valium. Karen spent a month in bed and couldn't do anything else without help.

A friend told Karen about an alternative health clinic she had heard about, Your Wellness Connection. Karen was ready to try anything, so she came to us at YWC. She began regular adjustments with one of our chiropractors, which significantly slowed down the spinning Karen was experiencing. We also treated her with cranial sacral therapy. After some time working on the physical body, we suggested she spend time with one of our counselors. Karen was opposed to it at first. She presumed she would hear everything she said just parroted back to her; besides, she didn't think it was an emotional issue. With our assurances that it was worth a try, she agreed. Karen saw our counselor once a week, in addition to occasional chiropractic treatments. Many of the exercises Karen did as part of counseling were about being able to see the good in herself and in the less than perfect world. After five months, the spinning ended; eighteen months in, she began to feel truly well.

Karen and her team determined that the vertigo and related issues were rooted in extreme stress. Karen finally accepted that she put that stress on herself through her own thought patterns and reliance on control and perfectionism. She would get easily angered if something went a different way than she had intended it. She held onto that anger and tightness inward, with little outward expression. She experienced this strain of control and the need to make sure everything was perfect both at work and at home with her family. Through her work with our counselor, she could let it go and not need the same control. Karen learned that everyone has their own journey to walk. You can walk alongside and support them, but you can't take the journey for them (a particularly tough lesson regarding parenting her children). She noticed that if she allowed her old thought patterns to come forward again the sense of vertigo would return.

Karen also had a complete shift in the importance of self-care, trusting her own intuition, and realigning with her spirit. She lives a calm life, not quick to react. She is now teaching her daughters to feel their spirit and not live in ego. Karen, like all of us, continues to work on her mind-body-spirit harmony and well-being. She has found balance and no longer lives in a world of all or nothing, black and white. She has shifted her entire life, including her career.

During her healing process at YWC, Karen was connected to a form of ancient Hawaiian massage called Lomi Lomi. Fascinated, she went to a class to learn as a practitioner. Lomi Lomi can release a lot of stuck emotions from the body, which Karen experienced. Once the class was complete, this former mortgage closer decided to shift careers and become a massage therapist. She went to massage therapy school for certification and is now an independent practitioner. Karen's desire is to help others find the balance and healing she has found on this journey.

Karen's...

Why: For grounding and balance to move forward through life with strength.

Intention: Facilitate healing and grounding for others.

Path: Be kind to myself and take care of myself.

Tribe: YWC team, Lomi Lomi colleagues, my husband.

Jeanette Jayne

Divorced from a twenty-year marriage to an alcoholic, Jeanette Jayne found herself extremely unhealthy, tumbling through several illnesses, on eight separate medications, very overweight, with high blood pressure, ulcerative colitis, asthma, high cholesterol and a recent diabetic. She had even experienced a TIA, or mini-stroke. Jeanette had been in counseling over a few years to figure out what was going on at home in the latter part of her marriage. In addition to her own health issues, she was handling a heart condition with which her seventeen year-old had been diagnosed. Jeanette's health was spiraling.

Lee, her business partner of sixteen years and dear friend, suggested that Jeanette pay more attention to her own health and well-being. He steered her toward Your Wellness Connection and me. I worked with Jeanette to determine a plan that would get her on a path toward wellness, get her off most of her medications, help her lose weight and gain a sense of well-being. We began with helping her body feel better through chiropractic care. With a little time and consultation with her physician, Jeanette stopped her antidepressants and hormone replacement therapy. Within six months, Jeanette lost 15 pounds and had more energy. Granted she now felt everything, the good and the bad, but through positive affirmations, a support system and reconnection to her faith, Jeanette was able to get past the bad. We made alterations to Jeanette's diet. As she continued to lose weight she was able to get off her diabetic medication and manage it with diet. She expanded her wellness tools by adding acupuncture, counseling and massage therapy. Her energy and health were better than ever before.

Then the market dropped. As a realtor, Jeanette's financial state was significantly impacted. Money was tight. She stopped coming to YWC and seeing wellness practitioners to save money…in theory. Her weight loss had stagnated. More importantly, she really missed the well-being and energy she earned by taking care of herself. After a year, self-care was important enough to cut back in other areas in order to afford it, even at a less frequent rate. What she realized when analyzing her financials, was that taking the medications had cost her over $300 per month. Investing in alternative ongoing care helped her get down to $30 per month on prescriptions and she felt a ton better - a much better investment, indeed. It was time to go back to her wellness plan.

As Jeanette began taking care of herself again, she lost thirty pounds. She still was having difficulties reducing her blood pressure so I sent her to an holistic physician, Dr. Suzanne Rowden. Tests confirmed that she had an overgrowth of candida yeast throughout her body. With a significant change in diet – gluten, dairy and sugar free – Jeannette made another leap to capture health. Jeannette remarried to a man who is a tremendous support. He cooks and maintains the same lifestyle that Jeannette has accepted. A total of forty pounds down and on only one medication (for ulcerative colitis), she feels great! Now, if she has a flare-up of her colitis, she chooses naturopathic methods instead of heavy pharma.

Jeanette's...

Why: Want to be a healthy, vibrant grandma and mom.

Intention: This is my way of life, a mindset of prevention and gratitude.

Path: Maintenance and continued growth; teach my family and share my story with others.

Tribe: YWC team, Dr. Rowden, my husband and children, my team at the office and friends.

Joni Rogers

Joni Rogers is an athlete and dancer who, like many of us, let that part of her life drop off as marriage, children and career came into play. She was overweight, yet still somewhat active; you could frequently find her on a tennis court. Joni knew she wasn't at her best, on the court or in any aspect of her health and well-being. One day a friend called announcing she was going to participate in a local mini-triathlon and wanted Joni to join her. Swim 500 meters, then bike 10 miles and end with a 5k run? "Could I seriously do that," Joni questioned? She said 'yes' to support her friend's goal.

When she said yes, Joni could only dog paddle in a pool, not swim 500 meters in a lake. The idea of the swim leg would wake her up in the middle of the night, heart pounding. She decided to tackle that first as it was the scariest. Taking it step by step she learned to swim. She had to learn how to bike again; but you know what they say about riding a bike. Joni was a little concerned she would bike so far out that she wouldn't have the endurance to get back. Training for the triathlon with her friends – now a group of over twenty women – they made it together. Running wasn't something Joni could physically do the first year. She opted to walk the 5k course and trained accordingly. Months went by and the group of friends, new and old, experienced in triathlons and novices, practiced together, checked-in on progress, and cheered one another on with words of encouragement. I was excited to hear about it from Joni and keep up-to-date on her milestones.

The day of the min-tri came. Joni swam, biked and walked. She was focused, having fun, exhausted, sweaty, and sore. I was participating in the triathlon as well. I finished and jogged back to walk the last bit with Joni and cheer her on. She was deservedly proud with a deeply penetrating sense of accomplishment. She did it! Her tribe all gathered together in celebration, with hugs and joy, excited for what they had achieved together.

Joni was able to take on a challenge that appeared insurmountable and make it happen with diligence, belief in self, and the love and camaraderie of her friends. She awakened the competitive athlete inside. She has continued to work-out regularly and trained for the mini-tri again this year. Her goal was to improve her time and run the 5k instead of walk. Joni is in better shape, lost some weight, and improved her tennis game. Swimming is now a form of meditation and gives her peace of mind. Joni has the confidence that comes with knowing she conquered something that felt overwhelming. She is living as a great example for her children being an active mom. Now there is an entire group of people with whom she has a new solidarity focused on healthy living. Most importantly, Joni is on a great path in a new wellness journey.

Joni's...

Why: Want to live for my family, kids, and be a good example.

Intention: Be a healthy, fit person in all areas of my life.

Path: Make healthy choices and keep exercise in my life.

Tribe: Friends and work-out buddies.

Jeanne Johnson

Abused child. Teenage mom. Cancer survivor. Divorcee. Multi-million dollar, multi-business entrepreneur. Highly recruited technology guru. These could be the chapter headings for the difficulties and triumphs of my friend, Jeanne Johnson. When she was legally old enough, Jeanne rescued her younger siblings from life with their alcoholic and violent father. She became pregnant at eighteen and shortly thereafter married a man similar to her father, as girls are apt to do. Over the next seventeen years of less than wedded bliss, Jeanne reared three wonderful children and survived cervical cancer before divorcing her husband, whom had already left the home. While strong, so much of Jeanne's identity and actions were born out of trying to meet others' expectations, be it for love or survival.

Post-divorce, Jeanne packed up the children and moved to Kansas City to start a new life with a new job, in a new city. Brilliant and bold, it wasn't long before Jeanne experienced success for the first time. She celebrated by buying her first home. A few years later, in the early 2000s, Jeanne took her tech savvy to new heights. Selling the house, she started a technology company specializing in remote access consulting. It was a million dollar company in less than nine months. Seven years later she sold it for millions. Jeanne beat her past and had life figured out, by all outward accounts. Yet that was not truly the case.

Life for Jeanne was about proving she could do it, that she could survive and thrive on her own and for her family. Financially and in her career she was certainly succeeding. She had made it, yet wasn't happy; she was surprised she wasn't happy. She began clinging to her children. Jeanne found herself crying frequently for no apparent reason. She cringed at silence because it was quickly filled with doubts, worries, and negative tapes running through her mind. The inner voice that celebrated her talent and victories was drowned out by the voices of self-doubt and unworthiness.

Jeanne first came to see me with pain in her right shoulder. We hadn't begun the physical examination part of the assessment and she began crying. Our conversation led to the suggestion of massage, sleep, improved nutrition, meditation, and water, all of which would rejuvenate the mind-body-spirit as well as help release toxins and stuck emotions. She took most of my prescription and showed improvement. However, Jeanne was not interested in being quiet and alone with her thoughts. I encouraged her to go through the Hoffman Process. She wasn't ready for that at first.

Each of us is on our own path and will address our issues at the time that is right for us. Jeanne's path was to first nurture her body and seek additional support. Jeanne's year of discovery really began when she participated in Hoffman and learned to trust her inner compass while releasing the cluttering tapes of self-doubt and unworthiness. Jeanne found authenticity to be the key to happiness in her journey. Life was about being authentically her, true to self, no hiding behind a mask of success or whatever she thought others expected to see or demanded. She now had a stillness inside, unafraid of the silence as the pounding voices of others' opinions and expectations were gone. When you have an inner peace, no chaos in the world can flap you.

Jeanne's commitment to being authentically all of who she is reignited her desire to be an entrepreneur. She started her second business, a new software company that quickly caught the eye of one of the top software companies in the world. The Seattle-based giant actively recruited her away from her company. When she finally agreed to an interview she asked herself, "Which me is going to show up?" She told me that in the past she would have dyed her hair and tried to look younger, doing something about her laugh lines, and charm them with what she knew they would want to prove her worthiness (even though they were seeking her). Instead, Jeanne chose to show up as herself – a smart, fascinating, brilliant business womanpreneur in her late forties, carrying a little bit of extra weight, with white hair, and laugh lines that tell the story of her smiles. That's who they wanted; exactly who she is. Jeanne's path led her to know how to take care of herself the way she always took care of others. She realized that she doesn't have to meet others' determination of who she is; she just needs to be authentically herself.

Jeanne's...

Why:	Want to be in balance, know serenity, and be pain free.
Intention:	Live authentically; be as kind to myself as I am to others.
Path:	Give my body, mind and soul what I need to be in balance.
Tribe:	YWC team and the creative people surrounding me.

Marc Kaplan

Performing, being on stage was the only time Marc Kaplan forgot about the discomfort he had with his body. He is a musician, conductor, theatrical director and music educator. He is talented in a myriad of ways, yet he dampened how brightly he could shine by hiding behind the weight. Marc struggled with being overweight his entire life, along with his immediate family. He experienced a drastic weight gain in the year spanning 2003-2004. Like so many of us he had a crazy schedule of early mornings, long commutes and work days, followed by evening obligations. Marc's daily routine began with a bagel with egg and cheese from a fast food place for breakfast, a Starbucks latte and pumpkin bread on the drive to work, and cafeteria food for lunch – usually a sandwich with high fat deli meat and chips. The calorie count would round out with a fast food combo meal on the way home from work and bar food later in the evening. Yet there was no time for exercise in his schedule. Does all or some of this sound familiar?

A year later, as his waistline expanded, Marc was working on a musical, driving between Connecticut and Massachusetts each night. His schedule kept him eating the standard fare of fast food while on the road. He was increasingly lethargic and his clothes were getting tighter and tighter. Marc's brother was also trying to get a handle on his weight. Together they discovered a wellness center that promoted colonics, juicing and healthy diets. It was during this time that Marc became aware that he was an emotional eater, nearly at a level of addiction. He began participating in a support group for overeaters. Marc and his brother supported one another as they weaned off of fast food. It seemed they had found an answer, which resulted in a 20-pound weight loss for Marc. It didn't last.

Marc began dating a woman in New York. A year of traveling for a long distance relationship tripped Marc back into his old habits leading to weight gain, again. One day Marc was in a horrific car accident. He suffered life threatening injuries resulting in surgery and an extended stay in the hospital. Even though in pain, he was silently grateful for the jumpstart in weight loss the hospital stay gave him. Not too long after recovery Marc moved to New York to be with his girlfriend. The yo-yo continued with the move; he put on all the weight previously lost, plus some. He proposed in January of 2010 and lost 35 pounds by the wedding that fall, but promptly gained 55 pounds the following months. Marc felt out of control in so many parts of his life, or he just wanted to hide; he responded to those emotions with food. It was a cycle he couldn't seem to break.

Marc's wife had gone to Hoffman a few years before seeking female empowerment and love. Her internal shift opened her heart. She and Marc met three months later. He had heard her talk about the Hoffman Process many times and thought it may be a good way to figure out what was at the core of his issues with food. Marc went to Hoffman in 2011. He completely shifted how he viewed food and his body. He lost 50 pounds in the first six months after returning home and continued to move towards his goal weight.

Marc's life is different now. He has a set of tools from Hoffman he can continue to use on his wellness journey. He acknowledges that he has a food addiction, specifically to flour and sugar, and has cut them completely out of his diet. While for many of us, moderation works, Marc's compulsion requires him to eliminate addictive foods from his plate, and it works for him. He is active with his overeaters support group and works with his sponsor. The mindset shift was a critical part of Marc's learning. He approaches health and wellness as reaching a state of being based on love and acceptance, versus a set of rigid goals that must be accomplished by shame, denial and suffering. Marc now sees exercising as his way of reclaiming his body; he sees eating healthfully as fueling his body, giving him the energy he needs to live his purpose. His shift has had a spiritual component as well. He consciously asks Spirit for help and meditates as part of his wellness practice. He also simply stops to breathe, bringing him back to the present moment, especially during times of anxiety, and helping him make better wellness decisions. Day by day, choice by choice, Marc created and is living his best life and is more capable of fully sharing his gifts with the world.

Marc's...

Why: Want to live a balanced life for myself and family, and to contribute to my community.

Intention: Show up and live an honest, authentic life.

Path: Healing and forgiveness for my damaged heart; using emotional tools and the goodness of food and exercise to reshape mind-body-spirit.

Tribe: My wife, brother, support group and sponsor.

Jodi Hobbs and Laura Henze

It happens all the time. A car juts in front of you or stops short causing you to slam on the brakes only to be rear-ended by the guy behind you that isn't paying attention. That's what happened to Laura Henze a few years ago. She was checked out at the hospital for neck pain and offered muscle relaxers and pain killers. She wanted a solution that would heal, not mask the pain; so she was referred to me.

As you know by now, I assess and treat the whole person, not just the ache and pain that may have brought someone to me. Laura completed our new patient assessment forms; and we ran several tests to get a baseline on cellular health among other metrics. Laura was shocked when I shared that her results showed many below average ratings, essentially identifying her as relatively unhealthy. How could this be? Laura was slender, never had a problem with weight, and was rarely ever sick with even a cold let alone a major illness. She didn't drink, didn't smoke; she didn't do a lot of things that she classified as bad or unhealthy. What our conversation revealed, however, was a soda addiction, very little if any water intake, and although she wasn't a fast food junkie, Laura's metabolism allowed her to eat whatever she wanted, and so she did.

I treated Laura's neck injury with chiropractic. Then we worked on a few of her habits. The first thing that needed to change was getting the soda, with its empty calories, carbonation, and caffeine, out of her beverage repertoire. Laura slowly shifted from soda to water and green tea. It was difficult at first; the caffeine withdrawal alone was literally a headache. It is important to remember that even something as simple as removing soda or coffee is a detox to your body. It could be a rocky few days, but you will feel the benefits on the other side as Laura did. Laura paid more attention to what she ate as she learned about nutrition. She told me, "I've always been a very positive, even keeled person. Unless a situation was life or death, most things in life didn't faze me or push me out of my positive outlook on life. I knew that I could choose how happy my life was by how I thought about it and managing what I put into my mind. I didn't realize until I started working with you, that I could control how my body felt, how it responded, by the choices I made to nurture it. What was true for my mind was true for my body." Laura also shared that she always thought she was healthy because she wasn't overweight and she didn't feel badly or sluggish – whatever you are supposed to feel when you are unhealthy. Then she said, "I didn't know how good I could feel until I listened to my body and nurtured myself. Paying attention made all the difference."

Laura's partner, Jodi Hobbs, witnessed Laura's changes. Jodi had a difficult back injury several years earlier. She completed physical therapy for it, but still had a lot of pain even years later. She believed the pain was just part of how she had to be. She came to an appointment with Laura one day and learned more about the spine and how everything is connected to this information superhighway of the body. Jodi decided to try chiropractic for her lingering pain. As a new patient we went through the same battery of assessments and tests Laura experienced. Both Jodi and Laura were shocked to find out that Jodi was actually in very good health, especially compared to Laura. How could this be? Jodi is a social drinker. She loves to cook, and not so healthfully, for their five kids and friends. She was 50 pounds overweight and had little energy. Jodi had been concerned about her weight gain and energy loss, but figured she was in her forties and this is just how things are as one gets older. The difference was that Jodi is a firefighter paramedic. Even though she was overweight she kept to a solid exercise regimen at the firehouse. She may have an alcoholic drink or two off duty, but drank a lot of water as well, as she understood the importance of hydration for her job. While Jodi's overall assessments rated better than Laura's, she still was not in an ideal state of wellness.

A firehouse is a tough place to be. The days and nights are long and unpredictable. You live a significant portion of your life with this second family, more often than not made up of mostly men. While the team has to stay fit enough to do their job and be ready and alert at a moment's notice, the environment can still create a few bad habits. That's what Jodi experienced in her firehouse. She loved being a firefighter paramedic, but the drill of stress, poor food habits and lack of sleep wreaked havoc on her body. She also found herself emotionally on edge more often than she liked, simply because she just didn't feel well and lacked energy.

Jodi's path had to include doing what she could to get enough consistent sleep even with her rugged schedule. She shifted her nutrition along with Laura and their family. The entire family supplemented the nutrition of their cleaner diet with Vemma, a powerful liquid antioxidant. Jodi dropped weight, saw a dramatic increase in energy, felt her mood stabilize, and even felt more rested when she slept. Throughout this process, Jodi and Laura continued learning and trying new habits, such as eliminating gluten from their diet, getting rid of clutter in the house, and taking more time for their spiritual practice. They both read my first book, Wellness on a Shoestring, and took the course as part of their journey.

In addition to all the improvements to their own well-being, Laura and Jodi had a significant impact on their communities. Their family is friends with several neighbors on the block who noticed changes in Laura and Jodi. They asked what was different. Laura and Jodi shared all they had learned. The neighbors began incorporating some of the same changes into their families. As a community they even brought healthier foods to share at group bar-b-ques. The same ripple effect happened at the firehouse. The guys saw a difference in Jodi – how she looked, her energy level, how she obviously felt better. Jodi brought her new habits into the firehouse, especially healthier eating. The crew got on board. Two years later, the Hobbs-Henze household and their extended circles continue on their wellness journeys, making healthier choices, listening to their bodies, and spreading the wisdom of wellness.

Jodi and Laura's...

Why: To always have the energy and joy health brings.

Intention: Live simply and healthfully, sharing our experience with family and community.

Path: Very clean eating, being gluten-free and focusing on nutrition. Exercising for fun, strength and flexibility. Keep our home and lives clutter free. Sharing the story and all we've learned with our tribe

Tribe: One another, our children and extended family, Jodi's family at the firehouse, our neighbors and the team at Your Wellness Connection.

PART TWO

Energize Your Life

You may be thinking, "How can I start this journey and change my life if I don't have the energy to fully live my life now?" This section will address that question. The two complaints I hear most often from clients are back/neck pain – I am a chiropractor after all – and a lack of energy. Pain and energy are not mutually exclusive. However, there are numerous reasons for low energy – some are physiological and others are not. We live lives of speed, busy-ness and instant gratification. It seems we almost wear it as a badge of honor to pull an all-nighter, have a packed calendar, and not have time to read fiction or complete crossword puzzles, or _____ (fill in the blank with something less-busy people have time to do). I believe we have a rising epidemic of adrenal fatigue in this country. I see it in my practice. In our hastened lifestyle we seek out food that is quick and easy, regardless of nutritional value. We rarely slow down long enough to realize that the lack of energy may not only be tiredness. It may also have to do with the metaphysical side of energy in our minds and environments. The second factor for changing your health is to address what may be depleting your energy and how you can reclaim it.

Chapter 5

Adrenal Fatigue

fa ·tigue [fuh-teeg] *noun*

1. weariness from bodily or mental exertion
2. temporary diminution of the irritability or functioning of organs, tissues or cells after excessive exertion or stimulation

You just got clear in Part One about your why, intention, path and tribe. You are ready to embark on a new or rekindled journey to wellness! Just the idea of all the things you wish to alter in your lifestyle can feel overwhelming. Please let me reiterate, this is not a race. There are no deadlines, no pace to keep. You set the path and move along it at the complexity and speed that is comfortable, in a manner that becomes a joy, not a burden, and yields a healthier and happier you. Choice by choice.

Working with clients through the early phases of their journey, I frequently hear how exhausted they already are. The mere thought of exercise or shopping more frequently for fresh, whole foods, or other actions they identified would be necessary, was anxiety producing. They have had no energy to fully live their current life. How were they supposed to find the energy to shake things up and take that extra step? These clients weren't just tired; they were experiencing adrenal fatigue.

Although it affects millions of people in the U.S. and around the world, traditional medicine does not yet recognize adrenal fatigue as a distinct syndrome. I believe it is reaching epidemic proportions. This chapter will discuss what adrenal fatigue is, how it impacts the body, and how you can reverse it. Whether you see yourself in the pages to follow or not, it is important to understand how to support your adrenals and create sustained, healthy energy.

A Lot of Power in a Tiny Package

So what are the adrenals and why do they matter? The adrenal glands, part of the endocrine system, are about the size of a walnut, and sit above the kidneys. The adrenal glands have an outer cortex and an inner medulla, both of which produce and regulate vital hormones. The outer adrenal cortex produces the steroid hormones cortisol, aldosterone, progesterone and DHEA. The inner adrenal medulla produces catecholamines such as epinephrine and norepinephrine, more commonly known as adrenaline and noradrenaline.

The adrenal glands and the hormones they control have important functions. The small amounts of sex hormones that are controlled by the adrenal glands have little to do with reproductive function. However, they are an important factor for menopausal and post-menopausal women as they are a key source of hormones when ovaries are no longer productive. Epinephrine and norepinephrine are critical to your body's flight-or-fight sympathetic nervous system responses. They are what you need when chased by a tiger, or everything that you find stressful in today's age. They increase your heart rate, constrict blood vessels, allow you to breath faster and better, and they stimulate the release of glucose (blood sugar) so that you have the energy to run or fight. Aldosterone's function is to manage the absorption of sodium and secretion of potassium, both important minerals. Cortisol is a critical hormone that regulates blood glucose, also influencing carbohydrate, fat and protein metabolism.

The adrenal glands' primary role is to help the body adapt to stress. That stress can be emotional, chemical or physical; the body doesn't really know the difference. This is the same stress response you get when exercising at a level that increases your heart rate. It is the same stress response when you are at your wit's end with your boss or are feeling overwhelmed. Prolonged, acute illness or surgeries are stressors. Allergies and food sensitivities are stressors as well. Chemicals, such as caffeine, can induce the stress response. Sorry to break it to you, but caffeine doesn't give you energy; it activates your stores and depletes your energy, leaving you with less in the long run.

Stress is not a bad thing; it's natural. The body is perfectly capable of responding and providing you what you need in short bursts. The adrenals respond to stress no matter the source because their job is to help the body maintain homeostasis, or balance. The problem arises when stress is prolonged. If you're running at 90% capacity all the time, there is little left when a new stressor arrives. You are less capable of handling one more thing, be that another stressful project at work or something as simple as fighting off a cold.

Adrenal fatigue occurs when the adrenal glands' regulatory hormone function is below the necessary levels to maintain homeostasis, usually because they have been overstimulated. Overstimulation can occur because of an acute situation that causes extreme stress. It is more likely for most people that overstimulation is a result of prolonged stress having cumulative effects on the adrenals. As we have discussed before, there is a credit and debit system in the body. Prolonged stress without the efforts to reduce and recuperate will lead to an extreme debit in adrenal function.

As the name suggests, the primary symptom is fatigue. This is not the same as tiredness that can be relieved just by getting more sleep the next night. If you have adrenal fatigue you may appear and act relatively normal, but you feel unwell, tired and have a general sense of blah (that's a technical term).

Signs and Symptoms of Adrenal Fatigue

- Fatigue
- Headaches with physical or mental stress
- Weak immune system – get sick easily, have a difficult time bouncing back
- Allergies
- Slow starter in the morning
- Feel rundown or overwhelmed
- More energy after 6pm than earlier in the day
- Fullness or bloated feelings
- Crave sweets, caffeine or cigarettes (stimulants); crave salt
- Blurred vision
- Unstable behavior

- Get shaky or lightheaded if meals are missed or delayed (hypoglycemia)
- Irritable before meals (hypoglycemia)
- Eating relieves fatigue (hypoglycemia)
- Cannot stay asleep (adrenal hypofunction)
- Cannot fall asleep (adrenal hyperfunction)
- Impaired cognitive performance
- Impaired thyroid function
- Decreased bone density
- Elevated blood pressure
- Increased abdominal fat

The Pivotal Cortisol

While the adrenals regulate a number of hormones, cortisol is one hormone that is crucial and a bit of a linchpin to overall adrenal functionality. Cortisol has several functions, both protective and energy supplying. For example, part of the body's stress response is to create swelling and inflammation, particularly when it senses an injury or attack, i.e. allergies or autoimmune disorders. Cortisol's job is to minimize those reactions and serve as an anti-inflammatory and anti-oxidant. That's great when we're experiencing asthma, or are sick, or in surgery. However, when our body is continuously bombarded with things it considers dangerous, like toxins or foods that cause gastrointestinal sensitivity (i.e. gluten and dairy), it can respond with a regular release of cortisol. For clarification, you don't have to have Celiac disease to be sensitive to gluten. Most of us have food sensitivities even if we don't clearly feel a more violent allergic reaction. You can get tested for just about every type of food if you choose. Cortisol's anti-inflammatory nature is part of immune system responses, blood pressure, and heart and blood vessel health.

Cortisol also has the role of managing glucose (blood sugar) levels during stress. It plays a part in fat, protein and carbohydrate metabolism to maintain blood glucose (gluconeogenesis). Your body needs proper blood sugar balances to make neurotransmitters; therefore, cortisol management is critical to a healthy central nervous system. Without healthy neurotransmitters you can experience depression, anxiety, and fogginess.

My colleague, Dr. Brooks Rice, a fellow chiropractor with a specialty in functional endocrinology, shares the differences in balanced and imbalanced cortisol levels. "What should happen," Dr. Rice explains, "is that each morning your body naturally increases your cortisol levels to wake you up. Your cortisol will fall gradually throughout the day. Then, as night approaches and your circadian rhythm tells you it is time to sleep, your body will release an increase in melatonin. Variance in this rhythm leads to adrenal malfunction."

If you have low cortisol, which is hypoadrenal function, you experience hypoglycemic (low blood sugar) issues. You will have a problem staying asleep because your blood sugar decreases in the night, which in turn stimulates the adrenals to release norepinephrine/epinephrine as a stress response and wakes you up. This most often happens between 2:00am and 4:00am." Dr. Rice goes on to explain, "If you have hyperadrenal function, too much cortisol, you have trouble falling asleep. It can cause insulin resistance with a rollercoaster of glucose levels, and a body that consistently thinks it needs more sugar, which causes you to want to eat more sugar. That leads to another insulin spike and more cortisol release. A vicious cycle is created. Caffeine stimulates the adrenals which triggers a release of cortisol into the blood and sets off the same blood sugar insulin rollercoaster. So even if you're drinking diet soda to avoid the sugar intake, you can still be increasing your blood sugar due to the adrenal stimulation of caffeine."

Cortisol levels are related to thyroid function as well. The thyroid gland makes two hormones: thyroxine (T4) and triiodothyronine (T3). The thyroid gland stores these hormones and releases them as they are needed. Dr. Rice tells us that, "Too much cortisol inhibits conversion of T4 to T3. Most physicians will only check the Thyroid Stimulating Hormone (TSH). TSH can look normal while the T3 and Free T3 are low and Reverse T3 high, all of which impair proper thyroid hormone function." Adding to the negative impacts of imbalanced cortisol, this hormone is also toxic in high amounts to hippocampus cells, which are important in conversion from short-term to long-term memory. It may be why you are always forgetting your keys or can't remember why you walked into a room.

I encourage you to have your cortisol levels tested. You can test your cortisol levels by blood, but a saliva test conducted four times throughout the day is a better indicator of how your cortisol levels are managed. Your health care provider will look for unbound cortisol and DHEA levels (precursor to cortisol). You want to see that both the rhythm and quantity of the hormones are in the acceptable ranges for the times of day the samples were taken.

The Road to Recovery

Just as you didn't get to this point of adrenal fatigue overnight, you can't fix it overnight. Depending on the level of fatigue you are experiencing, it could take you three months to two years to recover. Once you recover, you'll want to maintain a more balanced lifestyle so that you don't fall back into the same state as before. The good news is you can rebalance and regain proper function of your adrenals. The exception is if you have done so much damage as to fully exhaust the adrenal glands, thus needing synthetic support. Only your doctor can direct you at that point.

There are five areas that will help you on the road to recovery and provide ongoing support for adrenal function. First, avoid foods and activities that stimulate the adrenals, including: refined sugars and artificial sweeteners, caffeine, nicotine, alcohol, foods to which you are allergic or sensitive, other allergens, too much exercise (overtaxing the body), anaerobic exercise, and inadequate sleep. Both Dr. Rice and I suggest a gluten and dairy free (or at least limited) diet because most people have a sensitivity to these ingredients, which in turn causes an abnormal immune/inflammatory response in the body.

> *The way you think, the way you behave, the way you eat, can influence your life by 30 to 50 years.*
>
> **- Deepak Chopra**

That leads me to the second area: eat a healthy, well balanced diet that also stabilizes your blood glucose. We'll expand on nutrition in the next section. Things to keep in mind when specifically trying to stabilize glucose levels, include: eat breakfast including a high quality protein; eat small meals and snacks throughout the day (not just when you're hungry); when you snack choose low-glycemic foods (low sugar vegetables and proteins); in general avoid highly concentrated sugars (including fruit juices); if you eat fruit, pair it with a protein. These are suggestions that I know work for most people. Yet the bio-individuality of each of us means that we need to listen to our bodies. Try what I am suggesting and give your body a little time to test it out. Then listen to what your body is telling you and adjust accordingly. As the body is healed you may want to go back to eating three meals a day. Start by eliminating one snack at a time. Continue to eat whole foods. Listen to what your body needs. You may always need several small meals, while others may only need three meals a day.

The third and fourth elements of adrenal recovery are closely tied – relaxation and sleep. Relaxation will help you manage the stress and sense of feeling overwhelmed as you continue to simplify your life. Meditation and breathing exercises are excellent relaxation techniques. They can be done as part of a regular ritual, or on the fly when you need to center in a moment of anxiety. You can find a number of meditation and breathing approaches in Chapter Two, Breathe Deeply, of *Wellness on a Shoestring*.

The fourth element, sleep, is critical. It may be difficult at first, both physically and mentally, to allow yourself to sleep for extended periods of time. You simply must give your body the opportunity to recuperate. You will need to sleep eight, ten or more hours a night for an ongoing period of time to fully recover. Eventually you will find that magic number of how many hours your body needs to maintain balance. The body really does keep track of your sleep. It knows how much you need and credits or debits your sleep account accordingly. You have likely been operating through deficit spending of your body for quite a while. That can only last so long before you're bankrupt.

I have had the good fortune of getting to know Dr. Jyotsna Sahni, a physician specializing in preventative medicine and chronic management at Canyon Ranch Health Resort in Tucson, Arizona, for eleven years. When discussing the importance of sleep in preventing and managing chronic disease, Dr. Sahni shared, "Getting adequate sleep opportunity is the key. You can't always make yourself sleep, but you can make sure you get up at a certain time every day. Pick a reasonable wake time and be consistent. Over a few days your body will show you how many hours of sleep you need and will establish your bedtime." You should honor your body's requests. When you are tired at 8:30pm, don't push past it and wait for a second wind. Go to sleep. Dr. Sahni also suggests that you create a ritual for bedtime. You do it for your children; do it for yourself. "If you create a ritual," Dr. Sahni says, "you create a conditional response that prepares the body and mind to sleep. Just as nature gives us dusk before dark, you can create a transition time from active to rest. At least 30 minutes before bed get off your computer and turn off the television. Begin to darken the lights in your house." You already likely go to the restroom and brush your teeth before bed. Add other self-care rituals that will support relaxation; possibly a bath with soothing scented oils, reading or prayer. I love my work and being present with people all day long. I have to tell you that by the end of the day I feel like I have all of their energy, pains, discomforts, both sad and happy energy, hanging on my body. Part of my bedtime ritual is a nice hot shower or bath where I can literally and figuratively cleanse myself of others' energy and go to bed refreshed and calmed.

Sleep can truly heal the body. According to Dr. Sahni, "Chinese and Ayurveda medicine teach that sleep has different phases for rejuvenating the body, mind and spirit. The time between 10:00pm and 2:00am is *Fire* time – stimulating and rejuvenating the physical body. The time between 2:00am and

6:00am is *Vata* or *Air* time – emotional processing and memory consolidation. This is the time when you reach the deepest levels of the four stages of sleep. You can't make memories without REM sleep." If you want to understand more about the critical nature of sleep, refer back to Chapter 1 in *Wellness on a Shoestring*.

Finally, the fifth element to recover from adrenal fatigue is engaging in aerobic exercise (versus anaerobic). Aerobic exercise utilizes fat burning for energy, whereas anaerobic triggers the body to utilize sugars for energy, which requires the adrenals to kick in and stabilize blood glucose. Aerobic exercises are those you can do for extended periods of time, such as walking, jogging, dancing, moderate cycling, and swimming. Anaerobic exercise is what you can only do in short durations, such as weight lifting, fast-paced running or cycling.

My dear friend, body-mind-soul wellness coach and speaker, Jill Tupper, long suffered with adrenal fatigue. Jill was able to recover and move into the best state of well-being in her life. Jill shares, "Most of us gradually fall into adrenal fatigue simply by not listening to our body compass. Like many, I had ignored the messages my body was sending. So many of us push past the tiredness and substitute natural energy with stimulants. We avoid sleep. We ignore thirst. These all put stress on your body, as they did mine.

"We often think that if we just sleep an extra few hours that we're good to go. That's not the case. It is like when you take an antibiotic when you're sick. A couple days into the regimen you feel better, so you stop taking the medicine. The reality is you aren't healed; it's just taken the edge off the bad feelings. The same is true with sleep. We overstuff our lives, calendars, closets, food, etc. When we live this way, it takes more time and energy to take care of all the functions of the day-to-day. I believe that the mindset of people that are exhausted is rooted in a lack of respect for their capacity. I know I struggled with that for years as well. If only I could do more, work faster, and so on. Exhaustion is not a badge of honor. Exhaustion is a result of over-functioners, usually coming from a place of having a big heart for others rather than to just do for oneself. Sadly the message over time isn't that you sacrificed for others, it is that you weren't worthy of caring for yourself. It is a destructive cycle. Yet the body, mind and soul are designed for both giving and replenishing."

Jill shared with me that she was beyond exhausted, thinking something was really wrong, that maybe she was seriously ill. She determined that she wasn't suffering from a major illness, but the exhaustion was still heavily prevalent. She started a sleep experiment. She slept as much as possible for one week. After the first week she felt like her body was made of lead. "I slept as much as fourteen hours a day for a full month before I began to feel some reprieve from the exhaustion," said Jill. The edge came off after another month. She continued extended sleeping for three more months adding in mild exercise and a well-balanced diet. Over time, she was able to reduce her sleep to as few as ten hours a night. This continued for a year.

Jill continued, "If I tried to push my body it would revolt. After the first year I was able to sleep only eight hours per night. In order to make this life shift, fully rejuvenate and heal my body, I had to learn to let go of a lot of things that I thought were oh so important. The intense healing portion of my journey took about eighteen months to two years. Now I can stay up late one or two times a week. I only need 8 hours of sleep a night but I still prefer and give my body 10 when I can." Jill coaches and teaches people how to move from "Exhausted to Energized," also working with anyone seeking body-mind-soul well-being.

If what you've read in this chapter sounds like the level of fatigue and other symptoms you experience, I encourage you to get your cortisol levels tested. Also, go back and look at your *path* and add in the suggestions in the Road to Recovery section above. You can reclaim your natural energy and rebalance. It will take time, yet we've already established this is a journey to wellness, not a race or a sprint.

EXERCISES

Whether you feel you are suffering from adrenal fatigue or not, we could all use less stress and better sleep in our lives. Try the following exercises in your daily routine.

Breathing

From *Wellness on a Shoestring*, "Breathe Deeply"

Master basic deep breath work. Because inhalation stimulates oxygen diffusion and exhalation stimulates carbon dioxide release, your basic breathing exercise will keep the inhalation and exhalation in balance. Breathe in deeply, expanding your diaphragm fully (your tummy will push out) and expanding your intercostal muscles (you can feel them stretch wider). Make your inhalation last three seconds. Then breathe out deeply, pushing the air all the way out (your diaphragm will squeeze upward, toward your heart, and your intercostal muscles will pull together). Make your exhalation last three seconds. Then begin again, with no pause between breaths. Hold your hands over your lower abdomen to feel the rise and fall of your belly. When you're practicing deep breathing, it can be helpful to visualize the exhalation as starting from the center of your brow and washing down over your body like a waterfall. Visualize the exhalation as the emotions or negative energy you need to release.

Downshift stressful situations by taking a few deep breaths before responding to the stressor. If you're about to walk into a stress-inducing meeting, stop just outside the door and take a few deep breaths before entering. You'll be amazed at the difference.

Bedtime Ritual

Create a bedtime ritual to prepare your body and mind for sleep.

30 minutes before bed I will prepare my environment for sleep by…

_____

_____

_____

I will prepare my mind-body-spirit for bed by…

_____

_____

_____

_____

Chapter 6

Food As Fuel

fu·el [fyoo-uhl] *noun, verb*

1. something that gives nourishment; food
2. something that sustains or encourages; stimulant

I admit it. I don't cook. Yet, I do love food. I'm personally not into a lot of spice, but I do appreciate food rich in flavor. I eat a clean diet now, gluten and dairy free as well, but that hasn't always been the case. As an adult, early in my career, I usually had a relatively healthy diet. I had always been athletic, and I was in a health and wellness profession, trying to walk the talk. Over time, I have had a significant shift in my understanding of and approach to food. I ate rather well before because the basics were simple: salad is better for you than French fries; steamed is healthier than sautéed or fried, and so on. What I have learned, both through study and just listening to my body, is that food is fuel and medicine. What you eat can turn your health and well-being upside down, or right-side up, as the case may be. I have a very busy life, just like you. I know that eating a clean diet greatly enhances my energy level and supports every function in my body. I can feel it. I want you to feel it too.

In this chapter I will share a few fundamentals about how food creates energy in your body, and the importance of having a healthy gut. I'll suggest a few changes to your diet. We'll also talk a little about the time factor – the fact that you may not feel you can eat more healthfully because of how long it takes to shop, cook and prepare meals. Let's get started.

Energy of Food

All things have energy. You are energy. The closer something is to its natural state, the greater and more pure the energy. That includes you, a human being. It also includes what you choose to put in your body. It can't be surprising that the life-giving energy in a basket full of greens and colorful fruits and vegetables far surpasses that of a processed food meal with a shelf life of two years. Living, whole food has a vibrant energy and can help create a healthier, more energetic you.

The Institute for Integrative Nutrition in New York teaches that the way a food grows relates to the energy it gives those who consume it. Greens that grow upwards, reaching for the sun, give a robust energy of expansion and newness.

Brightly colored fruits and vegetables that grow above ground on plants and trees provide lively, happy energy. Vegetables that grow close to or underground, like squash and root vegetables, bring a sense of stability and warmth. This is also in line with the natural growing seasons of foods (spring, summer, fall, winter).

The same is true for the animals we eat. We absorb the energy of what they ate and the conditions by which they lived. If you think of it that way, then it makes a difference how you buy meats, seafood, eggs and dairy (e.g. antibiotic free, cage free, grass-fed, or wild, etc.).

How Your Body Uses Food

The quality of the food you consume directs the quality of the energy you have. Your body, specifically your genes, releases the energy of the food. When you eat whole foods, especially plants, it is easy for your body to unlock the energy they've stored from the sun and the earth. When you eat processed foods full of chemical compounds you can't pronounce, preservatives, modified sugars, colorings and flavorings, your cells expend a lot of energy just sorting through and separating the nutrients from artificial ingredients.

Each and every cell in your body makes energy. They all use the same fuel – food and oxygen. Dr. Woodson Merrell, in his book, *The Source: Unleash Your Natural Energy, Power Up Your Health, and Feel 10 Years Younger*, explains the body's food-to-energy process saying, "When your body digests food, it breaks down every mouthful into glucose (a simple sugar) and dozens of other nutrients (vitamins, minerals, fatty acids, and amino acids) that it absorbs and sends into the blood supply. To oversimplify the process: the bloodstream delivers sugar, nutrients, water and oxygen to each cell, and your cells' internal energy factories (the mitochondria) then use the nutrients to combine the sugar with oxygen and create energy." [1]

The components of food that contribute to the creation of energy are macronutrients and micronutrients. Macronutrients are the elements that hold calories, such as carbohydrates, proteins, and fats. Micronutrients are essential to the body's functions and include amino acids, vitamins, minerals and a variety of other compounds that support genes and cellular function.

Empty calories that are nearly pure sugar can provide a quick jolt of energy. That's why you often hear of athletes eating a big bowl of pasta the day of the game, for example. That may be fine on occasion and when you're about to burn off a lot of calories. But, that is not how most of us are. We eat sugar-rich, high glycemic foods because we like them, and then live a sedentary life. Dr. Merrell explains why that can be hard on our cells when he shares, "A sugar (or glucose) molecule's usefulness as an energy source…depends on several elements: how quickly that sugar gets absorbed, and whether or not it comes with a posse of nutrients that help convert the sugar into energy and clear the cell of free radicals created by the conversion process. Eating sugar alone, say, in a doughnut, without essential nutrients forces the cell to use up some of its stores of micronutrients to convert the sugar into energy, and that sets off a process of depletion."[2] Eating whole foods as complex carbohydrates alone, or in a well-rounded meal, in the long run will set you up for sustained energy.

The body also needs proteins both for their macronutrient side and the micronutrients they provide as amino acids. Amino acids are important for building muscle and hormones, and as neurotransmitters. They also serve as a secondary energy source. However, most of the protein we consume in a western diet comes from meats that also provide unhealthy fats. I speak a lot about healthy and unhealthy fats in Chapter 6: Eat from the Sea and Enjoy the Sun in *Wellness on a Shoestring*. The fats that support health and wellness are monounsaturated and omega-3 unsaturated. These fats are in fatty fish, nuts, and olive oil among other sources. They are key elements in healthy cells. Your body will resort to using these fats as an energy source in an emergency. If you do just the two things mentioned in the last few paragraphs: move from refined, simple carbohydrates to complex carbohydrates, and from unhealthy animal fats to those from plants and fish, you will feel a significant increase in energy levels.

One of the reasons why I love Chiropractic is that it engages every aspect of how your body functions through the nervous system. The nervous system is the information superhighway. It isn't just about the physical feelings that might immediately come to mind, like the pain you feel if you burn your hand or pull a muscle. It is the way every part of the body talks to every other part of the body. It does this through neurotransmitters. Some of what gets transmitted is based on the information your body receives from the food you eat. Dr. Merrell describes it, "On a basic level, food is nothing more than a collection of genetic signaling molecules. When you eat a lot of sugar you signal your DNA to produce insulin. Tucking into a slab of… beef loaded with saturated fat can signal your DNA to create inflammatory molecules that among other mischief oxidize cholesterol, causing it to stick to the inside of your blood vessels. Eating fish signals your DNA to create anti-inflammatory molecules to prevent this harmful oxidation of fats. Every time you eat, you ingest substances that interact with your DNA, causing changes at the molecular level. If you want to tell your DNA to create more energy, you have to send the right signals."[3] For your body to make more energy available you need to give it foods rich in the real food materials that signal your body to manufacture clean energy.

> *At home I serve the kind of food I know the story behind.*
>
> **- Michael Pollan**

Nutritional Approaches

I have the good fortune to have a nutritionist and wellness coach, who is also a dear friend, on YWC staff, Shelly Murray, HHC, AADP. She is frequently cooking something new for her clients or a class, and I benefit from the leftovers as my lunch or take-home dinner. My family has started cooking more at home in the past year. However, up until this year we ate out at restaurants or at friends' homes frequently. When we are not personally controlling the options, we can still control what we choose to put in our mouths. Fortunately, my friends, who are my tribe, also do their best to eat healthfully; so we choose restaurants with healthier options or a gluten-free menu, and cook healthier foods when hosting one another for dinner. I make conscious choices about the food I eat because I know what a difference it makes in my health and energy level. I don't just know this as a health care provider. I know it because I feel it; I listen to my body.

Listening to your body is critical. Ignoring your body signals is partially why people get to a point of adrenal fatigue as we discussed in the last chapter. You can also experience fatigue because you aren't getting the nutrients in your body; not just because you aren't eating them, but because you aren't absorbing them. You need to support a healthy gut. How? Eat whole fruits and veggies for their fiber. Dark, leafy greens will help keep your body alkaline. Take a probiotic to balance the flora in your digestive tract. Also, avoid foods that hinder absorption, like gluten, dairy and wheat (while wheat contains gluten, these are separate issues). Both gluten (that you get from grains) and dairy coat your digestive tract and keep nutrients from being absorbed into your system. I'm sure most of you do not have Celiac disease, but many of you likely do have some level of gluten intolerance.

Modern wheat has been modified in such a way that it increases your appetite for carbohydrates (in this case, breads and sugars). I spoke with Dr. William Davis, author of the New York Times bestseller, *Wheat Belly*, who said, "Consuming wheat opens normal intestinal barriers allowing toxins and waste to seep back into our bodies when our system is trying to remove them." Simultaneously, the intestines are less capable of absorbing the good nutrients, affecting your energy and health. Also, wheat impacts your blood sugar more than you would suspect. As Dr. Davis says in his book, "The glycemic index of white bread [is] 69 [on a scale of 100], while the glycemic index of whole grain bread [is] 72 and Shredded Wheat cereal [is] 67, while that of sucrose (table sugar) [is] 59! …The glycemic index of a Snickers bar is 41 – far better than whole grain bread."[4]

Take Crystal Jenkins, LCPC, a counselor on my team at YWC, as an example of how eating wheat can impact someone. Crystal is very active and healthy. A couple years ago she went gluten-free, which significantly improved how she felt, her energy level; it even helped her thyroid function. When she stopped eating gluten she didn't stop eating grains or wheat. She got caught up in all the gluten-free marketing razzmatazz of bread products that still contained wheat, eating more than she had before. She started feeling bloated and her energy had the ups and downs of a roller coaster (likely blood sugar imbalance and blockage of absorption of nutrients). After reading *Wheat Belly* she eliminated processed food. Wow, what a difference that made! Her energy levels got a major booster shot, her blood sugar was stable, and the bloating was gone.

If you want to increase your energy level, I suggest making the following changes or enhancements to your current diet. Remember, I believe whole heartedly that the best way to make changes is to add in more of the good to crowd out the bad over time.

1. Eat more real food. Over time eliminate processed foods and food-like substances.

2. Eat mostly veggies, fruit, non-gluten grains, beans, raw nuts and seeds. Limit your animal proteins; focus less on meats and more on fish.

3. Minimize or eliminate refined sugar (that includes alcohol) and caffeine. Replace the false energy you get from sugar and caffeine stimulants with real energy from food.

4. Become gluten-free and dairy-free (at least limit dairy). At the very least try being gluten-free for a month and see how you feel.

5. Remove wheat from your diet (at least limit it). Beyond the gluten, properties of wheat can damage the gut, keeping your body from absorbing good nutrients.

6. Drink water. It will provide the hydration your cells need to function and communicate. Water also helps you crowd out the caffeine and other toxins you have accumulated through the foods you previously ate.

Shelly Murray, the nutrition and wellness coach at YWC that I mentioned earlier has a few additional recommendations. She suggests juicing – making healthy vegetable juices with a splash of fruit. She says, "When you drink a juice, you are consuming a highly nutrient dense food that the body doesn't have to work hard to digest and absorb. You are consequently gaining a lot of energy without expending much in the process." If you don't have a juicer, you may have a Juice Stop or similar shop in your town. Shelly also suggests that you eat regularly throughout the day. "If you eat smaller meals throughout the day," she says, "you maintain a level metabolism and energy, while putting less stress on the body. You also are not so hungry that when you do eat you just gobble up food and don't really chew. Absorption starts in the mouth with chewing."

I am a believer in the benefit of a good detox a couple times a year. Shelly agrees, but suggests that, "Eating a clean diet will be a detox for the body in and of itself. Going straight into a regular detox program could be very stressful on a body that is used to nutrient poor and heavily processed foods. Start with a clean diet. Consider adding a healthy probiotic to support the digestive system. Then, several months later, more fully detoxify your body with a 2-4 day detox program 2-3 times a year."

There are many different ways people come to the realization that food is fuel and the linchpin in your health and well-being. My friend, Tess Masters, author of *Healthy Blender Recipes*, had an interesting journey that eventually led her to be an expert in making healthy food tasty and easy. Tess's story begins with sheer exhaustion. She was completely lethargic and also had an excess of candida (yeast) in her body. She went to a naturopathic doctor who introduced her to the concept of food as medicine. She shares, "I have explored most approaches to nutritional eating. I first became a vegetarian. I then adopted a macrobiotic diet. I thrived; but after ten years, found it no longer sustained me. I also tried Body Ecology, and cherry-picked from the pillars of health and whole foods. Over time, as I explored different food combinations and fad diets, I came to understand the bio-individuality of food as medicine and as fuel. The bio-individuality approach allowed flexibility rather than rigidity, and allowed me to find the right balance for me. A key learning was how important it was to keep a pH balance that is more alkaline. That happens naturally when you eat a lot of greens and veggies.

"Once I got to a balanced bio-individual diet that worked for me, I started dialoging with others about my experiences. I added yoga and meditation to my life as well as considering thoughts on energy. It all added to my customized holistic approach. I decided to use "the blender girl" for my business as a metaphor of finding the perfect blend for healthy living in my life. What that blend is can change daily or weekly. I just have to check in, listen to my body, and determine the right healthy blend for me at the moment." Tess's top three recommendations from experience: eat greens, stay alkaline, and stay hydrated. Eating live foods is key.

No Time to Eat Healthfully

I know you're tired. Fresh food means having to go to the store more often. It means the food could rot and will have to be used, versus stored. You'll have more food in your refrigerator and fruit baskets than in the pantry. That means you'll be preparing food, washing veggies, and cooking meals versus popping something in the microwave. That equals time and energy that you just don't feel you have. I hear you. "Michelle, what are you thinking? I'm already exhausted. How am I supposed to muster the energy to do all of this?"

Shelly Murray hears these questions from nearly every client. I asked Shelly what she recommends. She said, "I have several suggestions for my clients. What works for you depends on your lifestyle. You want to eat more veggies but don't have time to wash and prepare them? Use the salad bar. Load up a large container of all the precut, prewashed veggies. Be sure to get a little bit of everything that you like. I would suggest keeping anything 'wet' in a separate container, i.e. tomatoes. You can go back to this stash throughout the week to top off salads, mix in eggs or put on gluten-free wraps. Use prewashed greens as well. Now you can find even darker greens in prewashed packages.

"Another way to save time," Shelly continued, "is to order your groceries. Many stores will take phone or internet orders and deliver the groceries to your house for a nominal fee. If time is money it could be worth it to you. Also, it is okay to order from or go to a restaurant. Just choose establishments that have healthier options and be mindful of what you choose. You can modify almost any menu item. Many restaurants also have a gluten-free menu if you ask. Some restaurants even note the calorie count on the menu to help in your decision making." Consider bulk cooking and preparation as a way to save time as well. You could cook a large quantity of brown rice, steel cut oats, or quinoa at one time and have enough to store in the refrigerator and serve as your grain most of the week. Make a huge pot of soup on Sunday and take it to lunch throughout the week.

> *A healthy outside starts from the inside.*
>
> **- Robert Urich**

Saving time and creating more convenient healthy meals were driving forces behind the launch of Tess Masters' website and cookbooks, www.healthyblenderrecipes.com. In our conversation Tess said, "I started Healthy Blender Recipes because I wanted to share what I was learning on my journey. Time is precious. I had to learn that resting and self-care were valuable uses of time. But I knew people didn't feel they had time to be healthy. I thought that if I shared my journey it would save others time and help them realize that spending time on food is time well spent.

"We are all so concerned about time. Changing your health and well-being does not come by way of instant gratification. It is an investment and commitment to really yield the results. That is what I experienced and know is true for others. But it is worth it. The time I put into my health now saves me time and earns me time in the long run. I look at it as part of my vision on this lifelong journey. I feel time expands when I'm healthy and energized and not sluggish or sick. We all have the same amount of hours in the day. When you choose to spend time day by day and year by year doing things that support your health and wellness, you are dissecting the pie a different way, with larger sections being full of energy."

Tess goes on to say, "What holds some people back from making change and listening to their body? I think it is fear; fear of changing tastes and habits, fear of what others might think, or how difficult it could be. On the other side, what keeps me motivated is that I don't want to get sick. I don't want to miss my grandchildren. I don't want to miss great changes in the world. I have such gratitude for the gift of wellness in my life that I'm willing to spend time on it."

Like any change in lifestyle, it will take time and sometimes feel difficult and require work to eat an optimal diet. I've shared my preferences and recommendations with you here. The most important thing you can do is try these changes, sincerely, one at a time for enough duration to feel a change. Then listen to your body. Create a bio-individual diet of real food that is balanced just for you and what works best for your needs.

EXERCISES

Instead of exercises, I'd like you to try a few recipes. I'm including some of my favorite recipes that will help you easily get more fruits and veggies in your diet and ramp up your energy. Enjoy!

Nutty Granola

Prep Time: 10 min.   Cook Time: 20-25 min.

Ingredients:

1 1/2 C raw, unsalted SUNFLOWER SEEDS

3 C Bob's Red Mill Old fashioned OATMEAL

1/2 C ground FLAX SEED

1 C SLIVERED ALMONDS

1/2 C unsweetened COCONUT

4 T organic ALMOND BUTTER

1 C AGAVE NECTAR

1 1/2 tsp VANILLA

1/2 C RAISINS

1/4 C GOGI BERRIES

Substitution Options: Unsweetened dried cranberries can be used in place of raisins.

Instructions:

1. Preheat oven to 300 degrees.

2. In a large bowl, combine SUNFLOWER SEEDS, OATMEAL, FLAX SEED, SLIVERED ALMONDS, COCONUT, and dried FRUIT of choice.

3. In a small bowl, combine ALMOND BUTTER, AGAVE NECTAR, and VANILLA. Mix well.

4. Pour mixture from small bowl into large bowl and stir until granola mixture is well coated.

5. Evenly distribute mixture on cookie sheet lined with parchment paper. Press mixture tightly down until fully compressed. Cook 15 minutes or when golden brown.

6. Remove from oven let cool on cookie sheet for 1 hour.

7. When cool break into pieces and store in a clean, large bowl.

Note: You can easily double the quantity of ingredients and therefore ensure there is enough on hand to snack.

Lentil Picnic Salad

Prep Time: 5 min.   Cook Time: 25 min.

Ingredients:

1 1/2 C LENTILS

2 T OLIVE OIL

3 T RED WINE VINEGAR

3 T finely chopped fresh PARSLEY

1 clove of GARLIC, crushed

1 C CHERRY TOMATOES, halved

1/2 large YELLOW BELL PEPPER

1/2 large GREEN BELL PEPPER

2 GREEN ONIONS, sliced

4 ounces of goat or sheep FETA CHEESE, crumbled

SALT

PEPPER

Instructions:

1. Cover the LENTILS with 4 inches of water in a large pot and boil until just tender, about 15-20 minutes.

2. Drain and cool slightly in bowl.

3. Add the OIL, VINEGAR, PARSLEY, and GARLIC to lentils and mix well. Refrigerate until well chilled.

4. Add the CHERRY TOMATOES, YELLOW and GREEN BELL PEPPERS, ONION and the FETA CHEESE.

5. Season to taste with SALT and PEPPER.

Quinoa and Spinach

Prep Time: 10 min.   Cook Time: 25 min.

Ingredients:

1 T EXTRA VIRGIN OLIVE OIL

1 large RED ONION, chopped

2 cloves GARLIC, minced

1 C QUINOA, soaked for 8 hours, rinsed and drained

2 C reduced sodium CHICKEN BROTH

1/4 tsp fresh ground BLACK PEPPER

4 C baby SPINACH

1/2 tsp SEA SALT

1/4 C chopped WALNUTS

Instructions:

1. Heat EXTRA VIRGIN OLIVE OIL in a large pot over medium-high heat. Add ONION and GARLIC; cook, stirring frequently, until ONION is tender, about 3-5 minutes.

2. Add QUINOA to pot; cook, stirring frequently until QUINOA starts to turn golden brown, about 2 minutes.

3. Add BROTH, BLACK PEPPER to skillet; bring to a boil. Cover pot and reduce heat to low and simmer for 13 minutes. Stir in SPINACH, cover and cook 3-5 more minutes until liquid is absorbed.

4. Season with SEA SALT.

Serving size 1/2 Cup

Leftover Quinoa Breakfast

Prep Time: 5 min.   Cook Time: 5 min.

Ingredients:

1 C QUINOA, cooked

1 APPLE, diced

1/4 tsp CINNAMON

2 T ALMONDS, slivered

1/2 tsp pure VANILLA extract

RICE MILK to thin

Instructions:

Put all ingredients in a saucepan over medium-low heat until all ingredients are warm.

Leftover Turkey Quinoa Salad

Prep Time: 25 min.   Cook Time: 10-15 min.

Ingredients:

1 3/4 C CHICKEN BROTH

1/4 C fresh squeezed CLEMENTINE juice

1 C QUINOA, rinsed well

1/4 C dried CRANBERRIES, soaked in hot water then drained and chopped

1/3 C RAW PECANS, chopped

1 1/2 C cooked TURKEY, chopped

1/4 C PARSLEY, chopped

Instructions:

1. In a 3 quart saucepan, bring CHICKEN BROTH to boil.

2. Add CLEMENTINE juice and QUINOA.

3. Reduce heat to low, cover and cook until QUINOA has absorbed all the liquid, about 10-15 minutes.

4. Fluff with fork when cooked.

5. While QUINOA cooks, soak CRANBERRIES in 1 C hot WATER until soft, about 5 minutes.

6. Drain CRANBERRIES and chop finely.

7. Gently Stir CRANBERRIES, PECANS, PARSLEY and TURKEY into fluffed QUINOA and serve.

Quinoa or Millet Cold Salad

Prep Time: 10 min.   Cook Time: 20 min.

Ingredients:

1 C QUINOA or MILLET, soaked, rinsed, and strained

2 C VEGETABLE BROTH or CHICKEN BROTH

3 SCALLIONS, sliced

1/2 C ROASTED RED PEPPER, chopped

1/3 C PARSLEY, chopped

1/4 C FETA CHEESE

3 T slivered ALMONDS

2 T EXTRA VIRGIN OLIVE OIL

2 T RED WINE VINEGAR

1 large CLOVE GARLIC, chopped

1/2 AVOCADO, sliced

1 small TOMATO, diced

SALT and PEPPER to taste

Instructions:

1. Cook QUINOA or MILLET in rice cooker with CHICKEN or VEGETABLE BROTH; cool when done. (Can be done on the stove top in saucepan).

2. Add remaining ingredients to cooled grain and stir.

3. Put over GREENS and add AVOCADO and TOMATO. Serve.

Millet with Black Beans and Vegetables

Prep Time: 20 min.   Cook Time: 35 min.

Ingredients:

1/4 C MILLET, soaked for 8 hours, rinsed

1 15 oz can BLACK BEANS, drained and rinsed (Eden)

2 T minced fresh GINGER

1/2 tsp SEA SALT

1 C VEGETABLE STOCK

4 SHIITAKE MUSHROOMS, sliced

1 medium CARROT, cut into 1/4 inch rounds

2 BABY BOK CHOY, halved

1/2 C RED CABBAGE, shredded

2 SCALLIONS, thinly sliced

BLACK PEPPER, to taste

SEA SALT, to taste

1/4 C SUNFLOWER SEEDS

Dressing:

3 T EXTRA VIRGIN OLIVE OIL

3 T APPLE CIDER VINEGAR

SEA SALT, to taste

Instructions:

1. Place MILLET, BLACK BEANS, and GINGER in a small saucepan.

2. Add 1/2 tsp SEA SALT and VEGETABLE STOCK. Bring to a boil, stir once, then reduce heat and simmer, covered for 15-20 minutes.

3. Allow to rest for 10 minutes, then fluff with a fork. Or put all ingredients in a rice cooker and cook.

Vegetables:

4. Steam SHITAKES in a steamer over boiling water, covered for 3 minutes.

5. Add CARROTS and BABY BOK CHOY and steam 4 to 6 more minutes. Remove steamer from heat.

Dressing:

6. In a shaker bottle add EVOO and VINEGAR, season with a dash of SEA SALT and shake.

7. Transfer MILLET to bowls and garnish with SCALLIONS and remaining raw vegetables. Season to taste with SEA SALT and PEPPER.

8. Pour dressing over top and sprinkle with SUNFLOWER SEEDS.

Peachy Millet

Prep Time: 5 min.   Cook Time: 20-30 min.

Ingredients:

1/2C MILLET, rinsed

2 C WATER

1/4 tsp SALT

1 10 oz bag frozen PEACHES, pureed

1/2 tsp CINNAMON

1/8 tsp ground CLOVES

1/2 tsp pure ALMOND EXTRACT

3 T slivered ALMONDS, toasted

1 ripe PEACH, diced

Instructions:

1. Soak the MILLET in water overnight or 8-12 hours; drain and rinse.

2. Add 2 C WATER to saucepan and bring to boil.

3. Add MILLET, PEACHES, CINNAMON, CLOVES, ALMOND EXTRACT and SALT; bring back to a boil.

4. Reduce heat and let the MILLET simmer about 15-25 minutes until tender and water is absorbed.

5. Add in slivered ALMONDS and gently stir, divide into two bowls and serve.

Buckwheat Breakfast

Ingredients:

1 C BUCKWHEAT, cooked (as you would rice)

1 ripe PEAR, diced

1/4 tsp CINNAMON

2 T PECANS, chopped

RICE MILK to thin

Instructions:

Place all ingredients in saucepan over medium-low heat until all ingredients are warm

Cherry Bomb Smoothie

Ingredients:

2 C WATER

Half of 10-ounce package FROZEN CHERRIES (pitted)

1 CLEMENTINE, peeled

1 APPLE, cored and cubed

1 BANANA

Half of 1 bunch KALE leaves

1 T FLAXSEED, ground

Instructions:

Put all ingredients in a high-power blender and blend until smooth.

Raspberry-Pear Green Smoothie

Ingredients:

2 C WATER

1 fresh PEAR, cored, cubed

Half of 10-ounce bag FROZEN RASPBERRIES

1 BANANA

1 ORANGE, peeled

1 T soaked CHIA SEEDS

3–4 COLLARD GREENS

Instructions:

Put all ingredients in a high-power blender and blend until smooth.

Blueberry and Peach Green Smoothie

Ingredients:

2 C WATER

10-ounce bag FROZEN BLUEBERRIES

1 fresh PEACH, pitted, cubed

1 BANANA

1 DATE, pitted

1–2 heads BABY BOK CHOY

1 T unhulled SESAME SEEDS

Instructions:

Put all ingredients in a high-power blender and blend until smooth.

Veg Shred

Ingredients:

Include a handful of any of the following vegetables:

Kale

Swiss chard

Collard greens

Dandelion greens

Beets

Beet greens

Broccoli

Cauliflower

Carrots

Celery

Cabbage (red or green)

Parsley

Radish (any variety)

Turnip

This recipe can be made to fit your tastes. If you are new to veggies, try it with a couple of your favorites and then add a new veggie each time you make it. You can use three or four of the listed veggies or all of them. The taste will change every time you make it, depending on the ingredients and amounts you use.

Instructions:

1. Dry the greens in a salad spinner or let them air dry with a paper towel. (It is important that the veggies are dry before you begin to process them.)

2. Using a seven-cup food processor, attach the chopping blade and chop all the leafy greens. You may have to do this in batches. Put the chopped greens in a bowl.

3. Change the blade to a grater.

4. One by one, feed all the other vegetables through the processor's chute until finished. Add these vegetables to the bowl and mix with the greens.

5. Store the finished Veg Shred in an airtight container (glass or stainless steel). It will keep fresh in the refrigerator for up to five days. Save "wet" veggies (such as tomatoes, zucchini or cucumbers) as toppers; do not include them in the mix because they will make the Veg Shred soggy and it won't keep as long.

When you're ready to eat the Veg Shred, get creative. Pull out one to two cups of the mix and top it with beans, goat cheese, tomatoes, sprouts, nuts, seeds, dried cranberries, raisins — whatever strikes your fancy — and the dressing of your choice. You can also toss the Veg Shred in with eggs to make a power-packed omelet; or try adding it to soup or a stir-fry. Have fun with it!

Chapter 7

Energy and Energy

en ·er ·gy [en-er-jee] *noun*

1. the capacity for vigorous activity; available power

2. an adequate or abundant amount of such power

The energy around you influences the energy you have available to exert. Yes, the physical elements of your life are the primary source of your exhaustion and lack of energy. We've discussed some of the main culprits: stress, lack of sleep, improper nutrition, caffeine, sedentary lifestyle, imbalanced hormones, and all of the related syndromes and maladies that spring forth. There is a third perspective I'd like you consider when energizing your life – energy itself.

I speak frequently about energy throughout this book, particularly in Part 1: Plan Your Path, while discussing the Energetic Quadrant. I also share quite a bit about it in *Wellness on a Shoestring*, especially Chapter 4: Free Your Space. Therefore, I don't want to be too repetitive here, but encourage you to reread those sections for more detail. I know from personal experience the effect of negative energies (physics and metaphysics) on the energy of your mind-body-spirit. Even if you eat well as we talked about in the last chapter, you manage stress and sleep well, and you are not suffering from Adrenal Fatigue, you can still feel less than energetic. It is the influence of energy on your energy. The energy I'm talking about is the life force that is both physical and metaphysical. It is influenced by your thoughts, feelings and actions.

Clutter

The energy flow in your spaces may be hindered by clutter. I'm referencing the mental/emotional, physical and environmental spaces you occupy. What clutter is taking up space in your heart and mind? It may look and sound like self-doubt or the chatter of your parents, teachers, or bullies, anyone whose negative words still haunt your self-talk. It may look like the friend that doesn't have a positive thing to say about herself or anyone else. That is mental and emotional clutter that is dampening your energy flow.

What clutter is in your environment? Yes, I am talking about actual clutter including that pile of papers on the edge of your desk, the mail in the corner chair, the overflowing laundry basket, the kids' toys strewn about, and the sewing project that has sat on the edge of the kitchen table for a month and hasn't been touched for three weeks. I'm talking about all of that. We all have it to one degree or another. Sometimes it is just a reflection of a hectic week, and it gets picked up and put away shortly thereafter. But if left and compounded day after day, week after week, and ongoing, it makes your home an energy black hole. It isn't just the stuff that is out of place. It is everything that never gets fixed. It's the wobbly door knob, the mud stain on the carpet, the button that hasn't been sewn on your navy slacks.

Again, I hear you saying, "Michelle, I don't have the energy to clean my house or work on the honey-do list." It doesn't have to be done all at once. It can be as simple as picking up something that doesn't belong in one room and taking it to where it does belong, because you're going there anyway. You could make it a game with your family and see how much you can get picked up, cleaned up, or put away during commercial breaks. Take just 15 minutes a day – instead of a weekend warrior approach – and see how much can get done over time. Check out The Fly Lady online who will give you a brief task each day to keep your house in ship shape. Also, consider swallowing your pride and asking for help. A friend of mine, Patsy, had a 'cleaning crew' of a couple girlfriends who had children about the same age. Once a month, they all gathered at one person's house with cleaning supplies and children in tow. The children played. The moms cleaned. Then the moms got some downtime as well. You could also just ask a few friends to give you a Saturday and make it a mission to bust through your home with rampant organization. And peace of mind may be worth hiring a maid service to do the deep cleaning once a month if not the weekly chores. There are also handymen, Mr. Fix-it type services that can whittle away at the honey-do maintenance list faster than you may imagine.

Clutter can also be the excess of stuff. Do you really need all of it? On the whole we are a society of overconsumption, which includes our stuff. We love to buy stuff for ourselves and for others. Look around the room you're in right now. What is the story behind everything in the room? See that green vase. Do you actually like it, or do you keep it because Aunt Gertrude gave it to you and she is no longer with us, God bless her soul? Who are the people in that picture frame? Oh, your ex-boyfriend and several people you no longer talk to? So why do you have it sitting on your bookcase? The memory of the moment in time that the picture was taken may be good; but every time you consciously or sub-consciously see a picture of people that are connected to hurtful or sad memories your energy is lowered. If you keep things that you don't really like or that represent something that is emotionally difficult, especially if you put them on display, you are just creating a minefield of energy zappers. I understand there can be both sentimental and less than positive feelings towards something. You don't have to get rid of it, but it doesn't have to be part of your daily life. I challenge you to really take stock of the things that surround you and how you truly feel about them. The things you keep must make a credit to your energy account; you need to have some positive feeling about them. If you feel neutral about something, consider moving it to a new home. Then donate, throw away, sell or store anything that does not need to be in your day-to-day energy field. You will be surprised by the difference.

> *The energy of joy is the most powerful force in the Universe!*
>
> **– Alina Frank**

Look and Feel

Have you ever walked into a store, coffee shop or someone's house and felt a vibe? That is literally the vibrational energy you are feeling and how it resonates with you. What is the vibe you get when you are in your own house, office, car or favorite hang outs? What do your best friends say about your home when they visit? If you can't immediately say that these environments have a great vibe then something is off. It may be clutter, but it may be something else. It could be the color, style and placement of the furniture and interior design. It could be the level or placement of lighting, or the balance of electric and natural light. Perhaps it is temperature or air flow that causes discomfort. The noise level, lack thereof, or source of sound may be the quirk that feels off-putting to you.

In the coming weeks, take a few moments to just be in each environmental space you frequent. Walk in your home (or apartment or dorm), into the entry, and through each room. Look at the colors that greet you, the pictures on the wall, the furniture, the décor, the amount of light or lack of it. Tune into your senses, including your intuitive sixth sense, and derive what, if anything could be altered to improve the energy, your energy. If it is a space over which you have some control, make changes as you can and notice how your mind-body-spirit shifts. If it is a space that is not yours to manage, either make suggestions to the owner or simply limit the amount of time you spend there.

Living Congruently

Emotional and physical spaces certainly can hold energetic sludge that drains the vitality you feel day-to-day. However, there is an energetic powerhouse that underlies our lives – congruence. Nothing is more tiring and destroys your energy than living an incongruent, unauthentic existence. Whew, is it exhausting not being myself! I know this is true from experience. Like you, I lead a very busy life with home, family, dogs, my multifaceted business, my incredible staff, several professional organizations with whom I am engaged, speaking gigs, taking care of clients, my spiritual practice, getting a work-out, and just having fun. My time is accounted for from sun up to sun down and beyond, six days a week, sometimes seven. Most of the time, I happily jump right into each day and have the energy to carry me through without feeling emotionally or physically like a wet paper sack at the end of the day. How?

I actively, consciously, make choices to live my intention and stay on my path every day. It isn't always easy and I haven't always been good at it. I've said yes to a lot of things that were not really mine to do. Do you know what I mean? There are a lot of things to do or think about that are not in alignment with your true purpose, your authentic self, or your wellness intention and path. Often, we feel we don't have a choice. In fact, we do have a choice. Yes, it requires more grace and time to change the course of some situations than others. It is a process; one I am still working through and is my greatest challenge. Yet, I promise, as I am finding, it is worth it.

When you spend time and energy – physical, emotional, spiritual, mental – not living your best self, your true self, you are living incongruently with how God designed you to be. And it is exhausting. It is difficult to say no. It is sometimes difficult to stay true to your core being. However, nothing energizes your life more than living in congruence, when your thoughts, words, and deeds are in alignment with the perfect spirit-filled being you are, and your deepest, innate, purpose, wants and needs. It all works toward your highest good. I do my best every day to live a congruent life and am in turn energized by it. You can too!

EXERCISES

Revisit the exercises in Plan Your Path on page 55 that relate to freeing your space. Review what you wrote then and add to or change your notes.

15 Minutes or Less

We all have a spare 15 minutes now and then. Look around your house, office or car. In the space below identify things you could do in 15 minutes or less. It may be to clean out the magazine rack and toss the old ones in recycling or straighten or wipe down the bathroom counters. The point is not that you create another list, but that you can recognize that you don't have to have an entire Saturday or even a whole hour free to make a quick difference in the clutter and vibe of your space. Note things you can immediately think of or see to do.

_____   _____

_____   _____

_____   _____

_____   _____

_____   _____

_____   _____

_____   _____

_____   _____

_____   _____

_____   _____

_____   _____

Now, put this book down for 15 minutes and do something to free up the energy of where you are right now.

Thanks for coming back! How did that feel? Great!

Living Congruently

Now, think about what you really want out of life, in your heart. Do those thoughts and feelings match what you are saying and doing? Are you living who you are truly meant to be? If not, why not and what can you do differently? In the space below take some time to reflect on those thoughts.

What I really want out of life, what is in the core of my heart and spirit, is...

_____

_____

_____

_____

How do my thoughts and feelings match what I am saying and doing – how are they congruent?

_____

_____

_____

_____

How do they not match – how are they incongruent?

_____

_____

_____

_____

What can I do differently? Where can I make different choices that allow me to live congruently with my purpose, my heart's desire?

_____

_____

_____

_____

_____

_____

_____

_____

_____

_____

PART THREE

Enrich Your Life

Your health and well-being may start with you, but they are bigger than you. We are not creatures of isolation. We are part of a greater whole. We all want to feel important and loved. I find it is a fine balance to be present enough with another person to see what's in their heart and love them up without sacrificing myself. It is important to realize that taking care of you is taking care of others; the reverse is true as well through the interconnectivity of humanity. Surprisingly the more connected I am to self, the more I can give and the more for which there is to be grateful. It is all about people. People have loved me up and enriched my life. Now, in this third part of the journey, I share how you can live an enriched life through community, relationships, gratitude and service.

Chapter 8

Local Action, Global Impact

lo cal [loh-kuhl] *adjective*

1. pertaining to or characterized by place or position in space; spatial
2. pertaining to or affecting a particular part or particular parts, as of a physical system or organism

glob al [gloh-buhl] *adjective*

pertaining to the whole world; worldwide; universal

It is said that even the smallest of changes in the patterns of the universe can set off a chain of events that causes a significant shift somewhere else in the system. It is called The Butterfly Effect – the idea that the flap of a butterfly's wings in Asia could lead to a hurricane off the coast of Brazil – or another example that seems equally unreal, yet true. There is also The Ripple Effect of which you've likely heard. It is like the impact that radiates from the epicenter of an earthquake or the literal ripples that graduate from the spot where a pebble is tossed in a lake. These are theories in the fields of complexity sciences, chaos theory, physics, and natural law that explain the way change unfolds in our world. I believe the same is true for how the health and wellness of our world will shift – and you are the butterfly or the pebble.

As I said in the Introduction to this book, you've seen the news and statistics and heard the political debates swirling around the state of health and health care in the United States and the world. This is not something that can be solved by political legislation. It starts with each of us taking responsibility for our own health and understanding how we can impact our families, communities and society as a whole. Taking care of you is taking care of others. It is another version of "Think global. Act local." Knowing and seeing how improving your own well-being influences the world around you is a tremendously life-enriching experience.

> *If you wanna make the world a better place, take a look at yourself, and then make a change.*
>
> **- Michael Jackson, "Man in the Mirror"**

Social Ripples

You are as local as it gets in the greater whole of global humanity. As you move along your path in this wellness journey think of all the decisions you will make and all the people with whom you will come in contact. You will change with each choice you make. It may not feel like it at first. You may not be able to see it in the mirror or on the scale right away or ever depending on your goals. But you will change, which in turn will change everything around you. The choices you make to live your intention and move forward in your wellness journey will impact how you eat, drink, sleep, socialize, and move, even what you buy, where you go, what you read, and so on. I know that to see the shift in my life all I have to do is live my intention, walk my best path, and play my best game. That is true for you too. Watch, you'll see. How exactly you change will be unique to you, based on the path you choose. There will be a shift in your own, personal patterns – a ripple effect within your life.

Think for a moment how your personal changes may impact your family and friends. If you are making better food choices then you are likely stocking the refrigerator and pantry with better food. You may at first make one meal for the family and one for yourself. Then you may slowly incorporate the healthier meal choices into what the family eats as a whole. If you're drinking a green smoothie for breakfast each day, try making enough for the kids as well. Sometimes they are put off by the color green, which can be overcome by putting it in an opaque cup. Sometimes they think it is cool to drink something green. You could give it a name, like Hulk juice. Tastes will change over time; what they aren't sure about now, they may request as breakfast in the future.

When you make healthier choices in what you eat and drink, you will likely change where you go out with your friends. It will at least alter what you order and how many martinis you consume. Your friends can't help but notice. Let's pretend that part of your path is to be gluten-free and as organic as possible. That choice may lead you to shop at a different grocery store or the local farmers' market. It will require you to experiment with cooking and eating different grains. You will ask the server at a restaurant to point out the gluten-free items or if they have a special gluten-free menu. You may start a gluten-free recipe board on your Pinterest page.

Beyond what you consume, the other changes you make along your way will ripple out and change your family and friends' lives as well. Part of your path may be increasing your exercise. When you identified your tribe, did you consider friends that would become workout buddies? Do you have a next door neighbor or spouse who will go for walks in the neighborhood? Or perhaps instead of family time being a movie and popcorn, it is a game of flag football at the park. As you move more and your endurance increases, opportunities to engage differently with your family, friends, and even new people to your tribe will expand and change. They'll get moving too, and who knows where that will lead!

It isn't only your family and friends who will feel the ripple effect of the changes in your life. You can have an impact on other communities as well. How might you be different at work? Maybe you drink water all day instead of a new cup of coffee every 30 minutes. Rather than send a detailed email, you walk across the building and talk to Jim in Accounting. Maybe you bring a healthy lunch to work or walk to the café three blocks away instead of pitching in to order Chinese take-out for the second time this week. Perhaps, instead of donuts for the team meeting, you bring gluten-free muffins, green smoothies and fruit. Freeing your space, you clear off and organize your desk each night before you leave. Do you think your team and co-workers would notice? Do you think some of them might follow suit?

Peer-to-peer sharing of new experiences and new information is the greatest influencer of change. That is only enhanced by the rise of social media in recent years: Facebook, Twitter, Pinterest, You Tube, and photo share sites, now even fitness share sites (i.e. My Fitness Pal or Daily Burn). Share your stories, articles you read, recipes you try, exercises that don't hurt your back, sleep positions that help you wake up refreshed, and so on. Lead by example. Motivate your tribe! You have a tremendous influence on your family, friends, and the communities to which you are connected. That impact will come quickly as they jump on board, supporting you right away. Or it will come slowly as you involve them in your journey, or demonstrate the changes you're making just by doing it. It may only happen once they see this isn't just a phase for you; it is who you now are and continue to become. Remember reading about my clients Jodi and Laura in the personal stories? Theirs is a story of a ripple effect – from their personal changes to family, neighbors and work communities. You can shift your world!

Environmental and Economic Ripples

We live in a country of free market capitalism, for the most part. No, this isn't going to be an economics lesson. That's not my thing. Yet we have to talk a bit about the simple reality of supply and demand. Why is it easier now to find gluten-free products in stores and choices on menus (supply)? Because people want it (demand). Why has Whole Foods Market grown dramatically? Why have conventional grocery stores expanded their organic selection and partnered with more local farmers and producers? Why is there a boom in yoga studios and life coaches? Because people are seeking and buying those products and services as they strive to improve their overall well-being. In Kansas City, where I live, there is an upward trend in local restaurants over chains and in those restaurants serving healthier and more locally grown/raised produce, meats and dairy. People want it and prefer it. My own practice at Your Wellness Connection has steadily expanded services to meet the growing interests and needs of our clients.

As society's preferences go, so will the producers, manufacturers, wholesalers and retailers. Yes, it is a bit of the chicken and the egg situation – advertising influences our decisions; and sometimes we don't even know we want something until we first hear about it. Funny how that works. But make no mistake, inventors, farmers and businesses will research, test, identify needs and follow early trends to be part of the wave, or create it. The other side of supply and demand is that as demand increases, so does competition. With increased competition, a.k.a. options, you get an increase in supply and usually a decrease in cost, not to mention improved products. So as your path leads you to new and different choices – where you shop, what you buy, how you spend your time, wellness services you seek, where you vacation, etc. – you will impact the economy and help shape the availability and affordability of better options.

Also consider that if you choose to begin eating more locally grown and organic foods you are supporting not only the businesses that sell them, but the original producers. More organic and heirloom seeds will be sewn over the less expensive genetically modified seed. Just as fresh, organic food and water are better for your body, they are better for the Earth. A reduction in the use of pesticides will help heal the ground and keep our waters cleaner – better for you and all plant and animal life. A reduction in processing of all kinds reduces toxins in the air, ground and water. Purchasing fresh, more local food (versus processed food) means less energy to process, package and ship thereby reducing the use of fossil fuels. When you eat more fresh food you have less packaging to throw away and the waste is natural and easily decomposed. You could even start a compost bin for your garden! Eating with the seasons means that you aren't eating summer fruit in February that was shipped halfway across the world, unripe and less nutritious, again reducing dependence on energy.

I know I'm oversimplifying things. However, what I shared above is nonetheless true. And while the examples I gave are dominantly about food, the principles are the same for other industries related to improving your mind-body-spirit well-being. Your purchase power – what you purchase and what you don't – has a ripple effect on the economy and often the environment, locally and far beyond.

> *Never doubt that a small group of thoughtful, committed citizens can change the world. Indeed, it is the only thing that ever has.*
>
> **- Margaret Mead**

Healthy You, Healthy World

You are creating a culture of wellness, first within yourself and then for your family and every person with whom you interact. You can influence your work, neighbors, PTA, Junior League group, bowling team, and the community at large. You don't believe me? Why do you think researchers and media outlets can study and write about the "fattest city" or "healthiest city?" Why can you go to some parts of the world and every other person is smoking, while in other cities you would be hard pressed to find a place to buy a pack of cigarettes? It is a wellness culture that has evolved over time. Cultures can change. You and I change our culture when we take care of where we are, right now in the present moment, at this place on our paths – how we care for our bodies, our minds and spirits; how we care for others; and how we care for our environment. Choice by choice, local action can create global impact. And it starts with you.

EXERCISES

Take a few minutes to think about how you can be the change you wish to see in the world. Would you take action as an individual with your personal choices, or would you get involved or start a movement on a grander scale?

I would like to see the world's health and wellness change by…

I can do my part by…

_____ _____

_____ _____

_____ _____

_____ _____

_____ _____

_____ _____

_____ _____

_____ _____

_____ _____

_____ _____

How will your wellness journey have a ripple effect on your family and friends? Journal some thoughts here.

Chapter 9

Relationship (As a Verb)

re ·la ·tion ·ship [ri-ley-shuh n-ship]

noun - a connection, association, or involvement.

Verb (according to me) - connect to, associate with, or involve.

Part of our life source as humans is to connect, to be in relationship with others. That connection to another is fuel for our soul, body, emotions and intellect. Some connections are brief, simple interactions with a stranger in line at the store. Most are with those whom you associate frequently, if not daily, and for whom you care, such as co-workers, family, friends, or a significant other. However, the most important relationship you have is with yourself.

Relationship is as much an action word as it is a noun, like love. While that may not be grammatically correct, it is in practice. Healthy, positive relationships with self and others require effort, awareness, consideration and compassion. Relationships enrich our lives in too many ways to count. Dan Buettner wrote in *Blue Zones*, "There are some things I'd certainly recommend for what people would call successful aging [or wellness]. One of them is, in fact, to have a sense of social connectedness. Most people enjoy the company of other people, particularly other people who they feel care about them. That seems to give you a sense of well-being, whether that raises your endorphin level or lowers your cortisol level. We don't know why. People have looked for biological markers, and they haven't been successful at finding them. But something happens that makes life more worthwhile. The days take on more meaning."[1]

In the Beginning

Our connection with others began before our birth. Crystal Jenkins, LCPC, a counselor at YWC that I mentioned previously, tells us, "Relationship is innate. Our very creation is formed out of the relationship of two other people. Then we receive nourishment and grow by the literal connection we have to our mother inside the womb. When we are born, it is the first time we are disconnected from another. What do we do? We scream and cry. Physiologically, that moment is to catch our first breath. However, our instinctive emotions understand that we are suddenly by ourselves and we start craving that connection again. We learn quickly that crying brings attention. We are swaddled and held, once again connected. But because that physical connection cannot be there 24/7 we learn to survive without it, becoming more comfortable by ourselves."

Our rearing focuses on development of the intellect with a nod to being emotionally "well adjusted." As we get older, we often observe or are told directly that shutting out emotions makes things cleaner, easier, more adult, more productive. We learn to keep our feelings close to the vest, we trust others less, and we depend on ourselves alone. In reality, the further you step away from others, from emotion, from relationship, the further you are from self. It is easy to think you can be an island and do life by yourself. You can't. You weren't divinely created to be in solitude. Even religious orders that take vows of chastity, silence and poverty still live in community. You were intended to feel, to love and be loved, to connect. However, before you can have a true and full relationship with people around you, you must first have a true and full relationship with yourself.

A couple years ago I attended a screening of a gritty documentary called "May I Be Frank." In short, it follows the beginning of one man's transformational journey from self-loathing to self-love. Frank Ferrante is the subject of the film and has since become a dear friend. The film begins as Frank finds himself frequenting a raw vegan restaurant called Café Gratitude. He quickly befriends the staff. Every day, customers at Café Gratitude are asked a provocative question. "On one such day, Frank is asked by Ryland, one of the servers, 'What is one thing you want to do before you die?' Frank replies 'I want to fall in love one more time, but no one will love me looking the way I do.'"[2] And so the journey began.

Frank and I spoke as I was writing this book. I asked him about love and relationships. Frank said, "Our reason for being on this Earth is to connect with others. In order to achieve that connection, we have to be authentic which requires vulnerability. Authenticity starts with self-love. If you can't love yourself, you can't truly love others. In the film I start out trying to change my physical health and appearance so that someone else would love me. I ended up healing my heart and learning to love myself first. When I see someone overweight, I see an absence of their own sense of divinity; a fracture in their self-love." Frank went on to say, "With wellness, the food [and everything else] is secondary. The real nature of wellness is about self-love, the relationship you have with yourself."

Life is about balance. The same is true for relationships. Crystal Jenkins goes on to share, "Too often we get caught up in an all or none mindset –

completely surrendering self and dependence on others, or total isolation and independence. The pendulum stuck at one extreme or the other is out of balance and not for our greater good. It is in the gentle circular motion when the pendulum falls to the middle that we find balance or the sweet spot of being in relationship with ourselves and others."

> *If you don't love yourself, you cannot love others. You will not be able to love others. If you have no compassion for yourself then you are not able of developing compassion for others.*
>
> **- Dalai Lama**

When you have a healthy relationship with yourself, you treat yourself with love. Love is an action, not just an emotion. As an action, you do things that demonstrate you love yourself. Think and speak kindly to yourself. Give yourself the nourishment you need with good, healthy, whole foods and fresh, clean water. Treat yourself with care, ensuring you get enough exercise and sleep and address health issues immediately. Have fun, play and enjoy life, even give gifts or pamper yourself now and then. Isn't this how you would care for and show love to a child or other loved one? Why are you any less important?

You are just as worthy of love and compassion as anyone else. The Golden Rule teaches us to do unto others as you would have them do unto you. I say do for yourself what you would do for others. It is just as meaningful an approach to relationships. Unfortunately, our society likens self-love to narcissism, as if you are "in love with yourself" or "full of yourself." We respond by being the opposite of loving to ourselves. We go to an extreme of self-sacrifice and sabotage. This again is an all or none pattern. Instead, find balance. Listen to yourself, your body, your heart, your spirit. Determine your needs and wants and provide them for yourself.

Give Compassion and Set Boundaries

Show yourself compassion by forgiving, yet learning the lessons. How you treat yourself reveals how others should treat you. Often our relationships with others reflect the relationship we have with ourselves. As you treat yourself with compassion, do the same with others. This requires boundaries. When serving ourselves and others with compassion, we stand up for ourselves, show and require respect and ensure we are on equal footing in our relationships. The boundary of compassion creates safety, love, and forgiveness without requiring ourselves to forget, which is almost impossible. Compassion separates the doer from the deed. When you have compassion for your loved ones, you don't have to love everything they do, but you still love them as a person. Do the same for yourself. You've made mistakes and poor choices – in life, with your health, etc. Let it go. Be compassionate and separate the deed from your value as a human being. Remember your wellness journey is choice by choice, day by day. If you try to live it without compassion for self you will get stuck, unable to move forward.

> *Use the 50/50 rule! Take 100% responsibility for your 50% of the relationship.*
>
> **- Crystal Jenkins**

Boundaries in all relationships create clarity. Love and interdependence do not negate independence. Jenkins shares that, "Boundaries remind us that we are only half of the equation; half of the whole of the relationship. That means that you make up and are only responsible for 50% of the relationship. Yet you are 100% responsible for your 50%. The other person is 100% responsible for their half of the relationship as well. Think of it as the fences between neighbors. You can walk all the way from the other side of your yard to your neighbor's fence, but you can't make them walk across their yard to you. And you can't hop the fence, take control, make changes in their garden or clean out their gutters. It isn't yours to do. That isn't to say that neighbors don't help one another; but there is a difference between lending a hand and taking charge. Honoring boundaries is respectful to self and others. It helps both parties take responsibility for their own lives." You can't force others to do or feel anything, and they don't have that power over you either. Boundaries put you in an empowered position to own your life. Again, it is about balance and the sweet spot.

Choose Your Friends and Be Present

The concepts we've discussed so far are true for all relationships: romantic, children, parents, friends, co-workers, etc. While the scenarios and details may be different, nonetheless, people are people. And to have healthy relationships with anyone, you must have a healthy relationship with yourself. You also get to choose the depth of your relationships (based on the boundaries you set) and with whom you will have relationships at all.

You can't choose your biological family, but you can choose the connections you have with each member. You can also choose who you consider your family outside of biology. You may not always be able to choose your boss or co-workers. You can choose how you interact with them, how you approach your 50% of the relationship. You can choose everyone else in your life, or at least the parameters of your relationship. You absolutely can choose your friends.

Part of a healthy relationship is complete honesty with yourself and with others. That does not mean that every person in your life has to be 100% involved in every part of your life. Refer back to the chapter *Find Your Tribe* in Part One: Engage. You already have many different relationships, communities...or tribes if you will. Most of them are completely by choice. Earlier, when you read about *Freeing Your Space*, you learned about removing and releasing the clutter that blocks the path to your mind-body-spirit well-being. That clutter may include some of your relationships. That doesn't mean you have to necessarily cut them out completely. It may mean, though, that you need to reevaluate, have compassion and adjust the boundaries. Boundaries are not all or none. They are balanced, flexible, transparent, and permeable. The future of most of your relationships is your choice.

> *Keep yourself surrounded by people you can't live without, not people you can live with.*
>
> - Unknown Author

You can alter and improve your relationships by consciously choosing with whom you spend time, how you relate, and by being truly present when together. Living consciously, being in the present moment is the center of personal empowerment. You can't change the past. You can't completely ensure the future. Yet you can choose every action and reaction in the now. This is true when you make the healthy choice of taking the stairs instead of the elevator, or eating salad instead of fries. It is as true when you choose to spend Friday night playing a board game with the kids instead of hanging out in four different rooms of the house. The same goes for staying off your phone, not texting or checking Facebook when you're with other people.

Being present to the choices you make for your health helps you make better choices. Being present when with other people, choosing your interactions and being in the moment creates better relationships. Play. Have fun. You can only play, be silly, cry and laugh in the present moment. It is the sweet spot. You are the most connected and at a point of strength. When you are present with yourself, usually through meditation or self-reflection, you can more clearly hear your spirit, your intuition, and God. Be present and in the moment in your relationship with yourself, with others and with Spirit.

EXERCISES

Take a few moments to evaluate your relationships and answer the following questions.

How would you describe your relationship with yourself? Do you speak kindly? Do you give your body, mind and spirit the nourishment it needs? Do you listen when your heart, intuition, and your spirit are speaking to you? Do you have compassion for yourself? Describe your relationship with self as if talking to a friend about your relationship with another friend.

_____

_____

_____

_____

_____

How would you like to change the relationship you have with yourself?

_____

_____

_____

_____

_____

_____

Think about your three best relationships with other people (e.g. romantic, family, business, friends). What is it about each of these relationships that enriches your life?

Relationship   Enriching Qualities

1) _____   _____

2) _____   _____

3) _____   _____

Think about your three most difficult or draining relationships with other people (e.g. romantic, family, business, friends). What is it about each of these relationships that they feel draining to you? What can you do to change it?

Relationship   Draining Qualities   Change?

1) _____   _____

2) _____   _____

3) _____   _____

How can you be more present...

In your relationship with self?

_____

_____

_____

In your relationship with others?

_____

_____

_____

In your relationship with God?

_____

_____

_____

Chapter 10

Gratitude

grat·i·tude [grat-i-tood, -tyood] *noun*

the quality or feeling of being grateful or thankful

Gratitude is central to an enriched and fulfilling life. It enhances other positive feelings and experiences like love, joy, laughter and fun. And it can reveal a glimmer of hope in even the darkest of times. Gratitude is fundamental to a joyful, abundant and well life. Unfortunately, all too often people feel or express gratitude only in the extremes of their life. They are so very thankful when things are going really, really well; or they are thankful for what is good when life seems bleak. These are also the circumstances when people tend to pray the most. There is nothing wrong with being grateful in these life moments. However, gratitude, as with prayer (or as a form of prayer), practiced daily and integrated into your very being, will shift your perspective and presence in the world.

> *No matter how bad someone has it there are others who have it worse. Remembering that makes life a lot easier and allows you to take pleasure in the blessings you have been given.*
>
> **- Lou Holtz**

No one lives gratitude more fully than my dear friend, Dr. Paul Jernigan, owner of Divine Love Heals. Dr. Paul and I have had many a conversation about the peace and power of being grateful. I asked him to share a few thoughts with you here. "Gratitude is where the heart and mind meet," began Dr. Paul. "It starts with a conscious intention to be grateful for all the things and situations you recognize in your life. It is in a mind space. The more you practice gratitude in even the littlest of things, it heightens your awareness, and the more it becomes part of who you are and how you are, from the heart. Your awareness becomes internal leading you to a space of gratitude, without thinking about specific things…just being. When I filter my life through a lens of gratitude it changes my perspective. I purposefully begin my day with acknowledgements of people, things, experiences, situations and feelings for which I am grateful. When the alarm goes off each morning, I hit snooze and spend that time consciously giving thanks. Beginning the day this way makes the next twenty-four hours flow."

If you read my first book, *Wellness on a Shoestring*, you know I speak frequently about being in the present moment; I've reiterated it throughout this book as well. We connect with our bodies and our spirit in the present. We connect with God in the present. You can also only feel gratitude and be grateful in the present moment. It can be about the past, the present or anticipation for the future, but the experience is in the now. Practicing gratitude brings you back to the present moment and a heightened awareness of your body, your spirit and your connection to Spirit or God. Dr. Paul goes on to say, "As you are more in tune with Spirit and living from that space God intends you to be, gratitude naturally flows. Being in the present moment, in alignment with who God created you to be, is living gratitude. It is a conscious choice to get there, both the path and the destination. But once you make gratitude an integral part of your life, it is not just something you do (be grateful); it is something you are, and a deeper connection to self and Spirit."

> *Gratitude is not only the greatest of virtues, but the parent to all the others.*
>
> **- Marcus Tullius Cicero**

Gratitude and Well-being

A life approach based on gratitude contributes to your sense of well-being. No matter what the circumstances, you can always find something for which to be grateful. Think of the Cratchit family and Tiny Tim in Charles Dickens' *A Christmas Carol*. They were financially poor, had to work very hard, and had little food or possessions, and an extremely ill child who would likely not see adulthood. Yet they were happy. The characters expressed gratitude for their jobs, that they were together for the holiday, for the food they had, and that Tiny Tim was well in the moment. Mr. Scrooge, on the other hand, did not have a grateful heart and led life overcast with doom and gloom, until the end. It wasn't just his attitude that changed, but the joy he felt, the spring in his step, how he treated others and how they treated him. For both the Cratchits and Mr. Scrooge, gratitude impacted their entire well-being. It is not a matter of good fortune, but of appreciation.

Frank Ferrante, who you met in the chapter on relationships, knows firsthand that gratitude is part of well-being. It was at Café Gratitude that his life turned around, after all. Frank's past included addiction to drugs and alcohol, and a void of self-love. I asked Frank why and how gratitude is so important in his life. "Without gratitude one can easily get too focused on the pains of life, be that physical, emotional or otherwise," Frank began. He went on to say, "Gratitude is central to sobriety. You have to be grateful for the simplest things to keep perspective and stay sober day by day, hour by hour. Quite literally, you may just be grateful that day that you have fingers and toes. As I began to understand and live a life of gratitude, I made it my response to my condition and environment. Even if there is something negative going on in my life, if I can mine a nugget of gratitude in the midst of adversity I have a shot at a joyful life. I dig for that nugget even if I don't want to in the moment. I do it, because I know that if I don't, the feelings I'm having can spiral into a further destructive state and it takes that much more effort to get out of that state of being."

Similarly, I believe gratitude is a meaningful tool on your wellness journey. We've discussed how making progress on your path is a step by step, choice by choice effort. As Frank said, that gratitude helps him keep perspective in his sobriety, so it can change your outlook as you walk your path. Gratitude provides perspective.

Take Morris Goodman as an example. Morris is known as "The Miracle Man"[1] and for good reason. Morris was on top of his game as one of the leading insurance salesmen in the world…the world. Life was great by all accounts. One day, while attempting to land his small plane, he crashed. His neck was broken at C1 and C2 vertebrae, his spinal cord crushed and every major muscle in his body destroyed. The only bodily function he could perform without assistance was to blink his eyes. Doctors doubted he would survive and if he did he would be completely paralyzed. Morris didn't see it that way. He thought to himself that he would one day walk out of the hospital; after all, he could blink his eyes. He focused on being grateful that he was alive, had good medical care, the love of family and friends, and that he could at least blink. Little by little, through visualization and the hand of God, Morris concentrated on and regained function throughout his body, grateful each step of the way.

I'm reminded of two experiences that quickly snapped me into a state of gratitude. Several years ago, when my clinic hours were still 7am-7pm, I was on my way into the office at dawn. It was that time of day when it was light enough to see, yet the street lamps were still glowing, illuminating the morning mist and shapes were still more shadowed than clear. The street I take from home to office is a main drag. As I was nearing a major intersection a figure caught my eye. It was a man, in a wheelchair, wheeling himself across this busy road. Quite honestly, I'm not sure if he wasn't a figment of my imagination, as I saw him so quickly. But the penetrating feeling of gratitude that washed over me in that moment was very real. What a tremendous gift I have to be able to walk, really to move as I choose!

Maybe because I'm a chiropractor I'm particularly sensitive to the gift of movement, but I was struck by another image just this last year. My tribe and I participated in the annual bike across Iowa called RAGBRAI. This is a long, difficult and often very hilly course that stretches clear across the state. Riding on this course I came upon a fellow rider, a woman with one leg. She was biking across the state of Iowa, up and down hills, on a 10-speed street bike, with one leg and balancing on her left butt cheek! Amazing! What a profound example of not only rising above adversity, but being grateful for and making the most of the capabilities she had.

> *I do because I can.*
>
> **- Unknown**

Often we get so caught up with what is going wrong in our lives, the problem of the moment, or that we can't do something as perfectly as we would like. It is like picking at a scab. You've had a scab before. What do you do? You pick at it. Instead of being appreciative of the 99% of your skin that is fine and healthy, or even that your skin is self-healing, you pick at the scab. That's what we're doing when we focus on what isn't "perfect." Have gratitude for what is good and what is working in your life. I find that gratitude gives perspective on your health and all aspects of well-being.

Dr. Paul believes that being in gratitude has a significant impact on well-being as well. He shares, "Because gratitude keeps me aware, in the present moment, I make more conscious and better choices in my life. My decisions are rooted in love and with the best interest of myself and others. Gratitude gives me discernment and helps me perceive if my feelings and decisions are coming from a place of fear or love." He goes on to say, "Having a perspective of gratitude about even the basic things about my health – that my cells work, that I'm breathing clearly, that I not only can walk, but run – leads me to take good care of my body, mind and spirit. I make healthier choices about eating, drinking, and exercising, and even in how I speak to myself with kindness." Gratitude is a mindset that provides direction and supports healthy choices.

Energy of Gratitude

We've discussed energy on several occasions in this book, so far. If thoughts are energy, then there is certainly energy of gratitude, and it is abundance. I'm talking about the law of attraction. There is a common phrase, "What you think about, you bring about." The law of attraction, in short, is that you attract more of that to which you give energy, in thoughts, words or deeds. If you focus on anger, sadness, fear, debt, pain and loneliness; you will attract anger, sadness, fear, debt, pain and loneliness. Fortunately, the opposite is true as well, and stronger. If you focus on love, prosperity, happiness and joy, you will attract more of the same. It is only logical that the things you want more of in your life, would be those for which you are grateful – grateful that they are in your life now or that they will be soon.

Dr. Paul reminds us that gratitude exudes positive energy in two ways. First, being grateful focuses your attitude and energy on the positive, what you want more of in your life. While the law of attraction does encourage that you seek what you want, you also have to be open to receiving it. The second way gratitude shifts your positive energy is that it opens you to receive abundance. If you are in thanksgiving for what you have already received, you are demonstrating the ability to receive abundance and therefore attract more of it. Dr. Paul says, "Gratitude is an active, not passive state. Some people think it means you are not ambitious, progressive or going after what you want when you're grateful for what you have. They think you're settling. That's not the case. Because you are grateful for what has been given, you are actively asking the universe, or God, for more." As I've heard Frank Ferrante say, "Gratitude elevates our vibration in the world." When I stay in gratitude, I am focused on all in my life for which I am in awe and appreciation; and being in that space only brings more things, people and experiences for which I am in awe and appreciation.

Gratitude is a critical component of an enriched, balanced and joyful life. It gives perspective, keeps you in the present moment, connects you to your mind, body and spirit and leads you to make better choices along your path. As you practice gratitude it will be less of something you do and more of just how you are, how you exist in the world. In showing appreciation for what you have been given, you say YES to receive more of what you want in life. Actively view and experience life from a place of gratitude and I guarantee you will shift your wellness – mind, body and spirit. And share it. If you are thankful for someone or something they did, tell them! Spread the joy.

EXERCISES

What are you grateful for today?

Think beyond your family, friends, job, house, etc. Are you grateful for the stranger who picked up the paper that fell out of your purse? Are you grateful for the neighbor who helped you do yard work over the weekend? Are you grateful for the gift of creativity or of an understanding of economics, etc. that you were given? Are you grateful for new opportunities around the corner? In the space below, list people, things, experiences, feelings, etc. for which you are grateful.

_____   _____

_____   _____

_____   _____

_____   _____

_____   _____

_____   _____

_____   _____

_____   _____

Now, I encourage you to keep a pad of paper or a journal by your bed. Every night or every morning, take a few minutes to reflect on what you are grateful for that day. You will be surprised how that brings peace, power and perspective to your life.

Chapter 11

Service

serv·ice [sur-vis] *noun*

an act of helpful activity; help; aid

This journey requires that you look at a lot of things in your life differently. Selfishness is one. You cannot live your purpose and give of yourself if you don't take care of self. When the flight attendant prepares the cabin for take-off, going into her spiel she always says that if the oxygen masks drop, secure your own mask first before assisting others. I know you have a kind and generous heart. I see it all the time. However, most of my clients who are exhausted or have chronic issues are those who give everything they have and then some to their families, friends and job to the detriment of their health.

Giving of self is wonderful and fundamental to an enriched life. If you selfishly – or self-fully, as I choose to rebrand it – give to yourself first, you are truly increasing your capacity to give more to others. Best-selling author, Lisa Nichols, says, "Serve from your overflow." It reiterates the compounding interest effect we discussed earlier. Any wealth manager would advise that you always pay yourself first to build wealth and leave a legacy for children or community. The same is true if you wish to build "well-th," give more and leave a legacy of wellness. If you realign your actions with your priorities in this way you will truly be capable of serving more, doing more and being more. So be self-full. Continue to build your "well-th."

Then you can more fully serve others.

Why Serve

Why serve? It seems like a silly and even politically incorrect question to ask. But in this world of constant demands on our time, talent and treasure it seems a valid question to ask and answer. The answer we were all given growing up is that it is our responsibility, the right thing to do. Perhaps, yes. But, why? Maybe we should start with what service really is. Service is love.

There can never be too much love in the world. Unfortunately, there are a lot of people who feel unloved, forgotten, not cared for, unworthy, or just in need of help. They may be in need in this very moment because of a particular incident. The need for love may exist in this part of their life because of circumstances – within or beyond their control. Many, unfortunately, live in an ongoing state of existence in desperate need of help or caring. There is no question there is a need for service, for love. Those needs are not just in developing nations and blighted urban cores. They are in every neighborhood, and at some level, in each person. We all need to be loved and to love.

So why serve? To love. Don't most core purposes come back to love? Don't most answers to the search for the meaning of life eventually return to love? Don't all major religions and great philosophers profess the root of our very existence is love? When you were identifying your *why* at the beginning of this book, ultimately couldn't you tie it back to love? Love makes us feel alive more than anything else. We all need that affirmation – that we're alive, that we matter, that we make a difference. What better way to be affirmed than to give that same affirmation to another through service.

In his book, *The Power of Serving Others*, Dr. Gary Morsch, founder of Heart to Heart International shared, "I didn't intend to start a humanitarian agency. I was asking the same question as … Tolstoy …: What do we live by? What are we here to do? I discovered what he discovered, that love for others is what we live by, and I wanted to give others the opportunity to do the same."[1] Heart to Heart International is a tremendous organization that provides medical aid throughout the world. They operate with, on average, only 3-4% overhead which is practically unheard of in the non-profit arena, particularly for one of their scope. They can accomplish this through scores of volunteers actively engaged in all aspects of the organization and its mission. As Dr. Morsch found, love for others is what we live by; and we can express that love through service.

Mother Teresa said, "We belong to each other." We are part of one collective of humanity. We are an energetically interwoven fabric that can be strengthened or weakened by the way we treat and serve one another. You never know how one act of kindness will impact that fabric. Did you see the film, *Pay It Forward*? In the film a young boy wants to make a difference by helping people. Their payment is to help someone else – pay it forward. As the story unfolds you see the connections and ripple effect that eventually lead back to the boy. The law of attraction plays into service as well. What you give is received. What you put into the universe is returned to you. Karma.

I believe that every person has four letters stamped on their forehead – MMFI – Make Me Feel Important. Never let someone's outside appearance or actions fool you. We all want and need love. We all want to know we matter, that someone cares. In service it is important to see people soul to soul, not role to role. We're all equals, just human, when we see people as their soul. When people are in my presence I want them to feel loved for the person they are in that moment, their authentic self. If you know me or have been to Your Wellness Connection you know I'm a hugger. My staff are all huggers. It's our culture. We hug every person we come in contact with, heart to heart. It is imperative to us that we serve everyone with care so that they know they are important, they matter, and they are loved.

> *In a world where there is such an obvious need for demonstrated love, it is well to realize the enormous power we do have to help and heal people in our lives with nothing more complicated than an outstretched hand or a warm hug.*
>
> **- Leo Buscaglia,** *Born for Love*

Another why is that service is a wellness practice. It will give you joy. Joy releases endorphins. Greater happiness, joy, bliss, and love should be as much of an outcome you seek on your wellness journey as strength, weight loss, improved sleep, etc. You will feel in your mind and spirit, if not also your body, the well-being benefits of serving others. That sounds like serving others is self-serving. If you're only serving others to benefit yourself, you won't ultimately receive that benefit you seek. The universe just doesn't work that way.

There are countless reasons to serve others. I'm sure you have the reasons that are most meaningful to you. Eventually, all reasons lead to love. Service is love.

How to Serve

I know. You're busy. The idea of adding something to your plate, especially something that you have to commit to doing on a regular basis seems beyond impossible. You already take cookies to the church bake sale and volunteer at the PTA. Doesn't that count? Absolutely. And no one is keeping score, by the way. There are just as many needs as there are ways to serve.

Before we talk about how, there are three important things I want you to remember when serving others. First, you can only truly serve from a place of authenticity. Your heart should be in it. Serve to give, not to get. Second, service is sharing. You don't lose anything by serving. Service is love and in this way love is like knowledge. Teaching someone, sharing knowledge doesn't mean you are any less knowledgeable. It is like lighting another candle with your candle. It only spreads light. Third, service doesn't have to be a huge gesture. Start with where you are and what you can do. The small things can be as meaningful as the grandiose. You don't have to change the world, but you can change someone's world, even if just for a moment.

The Starfish Story perfectly illustrates the idea of doing what you can. I imagine you've heard a version of this story before as it has become quite popular. Here's my favorite account as adapted from the original, "The Star Thrower" by Loren Eiseley.

> One day a man was walking along the beach when he noticed a boy picking something up and gently throwing it into the ocean. Approaching the boy, he asked, "What are you doing?"
>
> The youth replied, "Throwing starfish back into the ocean. The surf is up and the tide is going out. If I don't throw them back, they'll die."
>
> "Son," the man said, "don't you realize there are miles and miles of beach and hundreds of starfish? You can't make a difference!"
>
> After listening politely, the boy bent down, picked up another starfish, and threw it back into the surf. Then, smiling at the man, he said, "I made a difference for that one."

Does serving others mean you have to write big checks, or fly off to the location of the next natural disaster zone? Does it mean you need to commit to three to five hours a week to meet with your Little Brother? No. If you can, wonderful! Money is always needed by non-profits and even service oriented for-profit entities. Major disasters have major needs both in the immediate aftermath and for many months and years beyond. Some service works best through a relationship developed over time through committed and consistent efforts. If you can give in those ways, then by all means, do. Not everyone can.

Maybe you can't write a big check, but you can buy an extra canned good or two each time you go to the grocery store and drop it in the community food pantry's bin on your way out of the store. Maybe you can't or don't want to go to the site of an earthquake, hurricane, or tornado; and quite honestly, unless you are a medical professional, specialist or with an agency you shouldn't venture into such situations. But you can donate extra clothes, toiletries, food, water bottles and whatever is needed. You can always send prayers. Maybe you can't commit to a long-term, intense one-on-one mentorship or coaching a kids' sports team. You likely can participate in a community activity that supports such organizations, or buy a candy bar (one) when they're raising money for team t-shirts. The point is the scale of what you do and how many people you impact doesn't have to be the biggest and broadest gesture to be meaningful.

Not every act of service is part of a coordinated effort, part of an organization, a campaign to raise funds for xyz mission or even planned. You serve others when you smile. Just a smile. You never know when someone needs a smile. Whether your smile serves as just a little pick-me-up for the receiver or gives them the greatest of pleasures to feel acknowledged for perhaps the first time in a long time, it matters. Leo Buscaglia, a professor and inspiring teacher on love, tells a story about a young man in the depths of despair feeling unloved and unwanted in the world. He walks to the pier intending to commit suicide. He does and leaves a note. It says that all he needed to prevent himself from jumping was a smile, an affirmation from someone that he was seen. That's a gloomy thought, and I'm paraphrasing the story, but the meaning is still valid. While this story may seem an extreme example, service to others, even in just a kind gesture, demonstrates love and can mean the world to someone.

I have been loved-up by so many wonderful people throughout my life that served me and made a difference both in good times and bad. Whether it was the nun who made a little girl feel so welcomed and loved even though

I wasn't Catholic and didn't go to her school; the woman who made clothes for me; or the Lakins who believed in me and told me I could do anything as I got older. I have been blessed with love. In this moment I particularly remember my babysitter, Maggie. Maggie was very special. My family lived in California from when I was three to nine. Back then, my brother Mike, Maggie's son Tim, and I were the Three Musketeers. We had so much fun; Maggie made even walking across the street fun. She was a tremendous gift of love that has been prevalent in my life. We moved to Kansas when I was nine. Maggie sent me a birthday card every year until she died, which was about five years ago. She always took the time to write a little note on the left panel. It meant the world to me, especially as a child, but even as an adult. We didn't speak frequently and I probably only saw her four times after we moved to Kansas. When I heard of her death, I wanted to pay my respects to this woman with a servant's heart. The funeral was the day before the fall health festival my company hosts each year. So I flew to California to say good-bye and thank you, and flew back the same day. The message is you never know how you are going to impact another person's life. Be kind. Serve. Love.

There are so many people whose need isn't food, clothing, shelter, or money. It's human connection. This is particularly a need in the elderly population. Not everyone has a family full of kids and grandkids that call, visit, and do things together. Even if they do, holidays are not the only days people need love; and isn't that usually when we reach out? There is also a growing population of single adults – be it that they never married or went through divorce. It is easy to assume people have plans or are off living their life just because you haven't heard from them. That very well may not be the case, particularly as we age. You can serve by reaching out, inviting them, folding them into your family if they're close. You're probably great at connecting and being thoughtful with your immediate family and closest friends. You call them on their birthday. You check-in to see how they're feeling when you know they've been sick. You ask how their job search is going, if their Dad is recovering from surgery well, and so on. You ask if there is anything you can do. Consider doing the same with people you don't know quite as well. I'm not suggesting that everyone has to be your friend or that it is even healthy to try to be the giver of happiness to everyone with whom you come in contact. I'm only saying be aware, be friendly, and connect, when and where it makes sense and feels right.

There are so many chances to serve others, and therefore enrich your life.

Here are several ways to serve: donate money or goods, volunteer with an organization once or ongoing, serve on the board of directors of a non-profit, smile to everyone you meet, say a kind word to a stranger, drink a cup of tea with your widowed next door neighbor, or simply call a friend or your Dad.

Your personal wellness will be enhanced as service becomes part of your journey. Your efforts, no matter how big or small, will shift the energy of the universe and strengthen the fabric of humanity. And remember to receive is just as important as serving. Allow others to serve you. It can be difficult, but others want to help you as much as you want to help them. Being willing to receive a blessing from others is giving them the blessing of being able to serve.

> *Being unwanted, unloved, uncared for, forgotten by everybody, I think that is a much greater hunger, a much greater poverty than the person who has nothing to eat.*
>
> **- Mother Teresa**

EXERCISES

What bigger causes speak to your heart?

Is there a disease you'd like to fight to help those dealing with it or those who have survived, like breast cancer? Is there a part of the world you'd like to support, like the Sudan? Is there a particular issue that you care a lot about, such as hunger or homelessness? Maybe it is a broad, earth or animal focused cause, like clean oceans or animal shelters? In the space below write the causes, the needs that resonate most with you. Under each cause list how you would like to get involved. Be realistic about the time, effort and/or funds you can give. Then identify specific organizations that are local, national or international that may address that need. It may even be your kids' school or connected to your faith community or the charity your company sponsors.

1) _____ speaks to my heart.

I'd really like to get involved by

_____

_____

_____

_____

Organizations that do that include

_____

_____

_____

_____

2) _____ speaks to my heart.

I'd really like to get involved by

_____

_____

_____

_____

Organizations that do that include

_____

_____

_____

_____

3) _____ speaks to my heart.

I'd really like to get involved by

_____

_____

_____

_____

Organizations that do that include

_____

_____

_____

_____

How Can I Serve?

It is so easy to get caught up in our own lives, even if that includes taking care of things for our immediate family. Are there people in your life to whom you would like to proactively reach out? Are there people who may really need a friend, or just a friendly voice? In the space below identify who those people might be and how you can connect, e.g., *Person*: woman I always run into at the mailbox; *How I Can Serve Them*: say hello next time.

Person   **How I Can Serve Them**

_____   _____

_____   _____

_____   _____

_____   _____

_____   _____

_____   _____

_____   _____

_____   _____

_____   _____

_____   _____

_____   _____

Epilogue

Continuing the Journey

EPILOGUE

My greatest hope is that you progress toward and reach optimal wellness, mind-body-spirit. This book is centered on heart, because there is a difference between having knowledge of information and knowing it in your heart from experience. I wrote this book to serve as a guide on your wellness journey. I believe your journey hinges on three factors: engaging, energizing and enriching your life.

Engaging a wellness lifestyle must start by knowing your *why*, why wellness is important to you. Whatever your reason, it is likely rooted in love. Next, set your intention, the purpose and approach for your wellness journey. Plan your path, the actions you will take, the ideas that will direct the choices that you make to move you toward that life you are meant to live. Accept that wellness is a journey; be patient with yourself. Accept that you will most likely stray from that path, briefly get stuck or run into an obstacle. It is okay. Take your time. Enjoy the moments. If you wander off the path, just wander back to it. There is no benefit in regretting the past mistakes or seemingly wasted time. In order to make the most of your journey find a tribe of people that can teach you, take the journey with you or cheer you along the way.

I most frequently see clients for pain and exhaustion, a sheer lack of energy. Adrenal fatigue is nearly epidemic. If you are experiencing that level of fatigue there are things you can do to reverse it. If you are experiencing early signs, you can change course. Nutrition is critical to having the energy to live your life. Food is meant to be fuel. If you view it that way, you will make better choices. You wouldn't put tar in your car's gas tank; why put the equivalent food-like substance in your body? You will get the same result in your body as you would in your car. The energy and sense of vitality you have also is related to the mental, physical and environmental clutter in your world. Clean out the clutter, create a good vibe and your energy will boost. But, nothing zaps your energy like living an unauthentic, incongruent life. Become aware of living a life where your heart's desire is in alignment with your thoughts, words and deeds.

And finally, enrich your journey with love. Invest time and attention in the relationships you have with yourself, friends, family and community. You train people how to treat you by how you treat yourself. As you change, as you make different choices, you will create a ripple effect throughout your life and everything and everyone around you. You truly can change the health and well-being of the world! Be in gratitude for all that you are and all that you have. The more you live in the present moment and are grateful for everything, everyone and every experience, the more your life will transform and give you more for which to be grateful. Enrich your life by loving others through service. Be self-full so you can give more to others. I know the more self-full I am, the more peace I have in my heart. The more grateful I am, the more I live my life in the present. The more present I am, the greater the impact I can have on myself and others. I have an enriched and blessed life! You can too!

My wish for you is a wellness journey with a foundation of heart and energy of joy, enriched by love!

Hugs,

Michelle

ADDITIONAL VIBRANT HEALTH RESOURCES

These resources can help guide you as you continue your wellness journey.

Johnna Albi and Catherine Walthers: *Greens Glorious Greens: More Than 140 Ways to Prepare All Those Great-Tasting, Super-Healthy, Beautiful Leafy Greens*. New York, NY: St. Martin's Griffin, 1996.

Arbinger Institute: *www.arbinger.com*

Art of Living: *www.artofliving.org*

Michael Bernard Beckwith: Agape International Spiritual Center: *www.agapelive.com*

Blendtec: *www.blendtec.com*

Victoria Boutenko: *Green for Life*. Canada: Raw Family Publishing, 2005.

Brene Brown, Ph.D., L.M.S.W.: *The Gifts of Imperfection: Let Go of Who You Think You're Supposed to Be and Embrace Who You Are*. Center City, MN: Hazelden, 2010. *www.brenebrown.com*

Les Brown: *www.lesbrown.com*

Ciardha Carey: *www.breathmechanics.com*

Centerpointe Meditation: *www.centerpointe.com*

Centers for Disease Control and Prevention: "Eat a Variety of Fruits and Vegetables Every Day," *www.fruitsandveggiesmatter.gov/*.

Chicken Soup for the Soul: *www.chickensoup.com*

Sonia Choquette: *The Answer Is Simple ... Love Yourself, Live Your Spirit!* Hay House, 2008. *www.soniachoquette.com*

Maiysha Clairborne, M.D.: *www.mbswellness.org*

The Daily Green, "Top 12 Foods to Eat Organic": *www.thedailygreen.com/healthy-eating/eat-safe/Dirty-Dozen-Foods*.

Daily Word®: *www.dailyword.com*

William Davis, M.D.: *Wheat Belly: Lose the Wheat, Lose the Weight, and Find Your Path Back to Health*. New York, NY: Rodale, Inc., 2011.

John Douillard, Ph.D.: *Body, Mind, and Sport: The Mind-Body Guide to Lifelong Health, Fitness and Your Personal Best*. New York, NY: Three Rivers Press, 2001.

Wayne W. Dyer, Ph.D.: *The Power of Intention*. Carlsbad, CA: Hay House, Inc., 2004. *www.drwaynedyer.com*

Linda Ellis: *The Dash. www.lindaellis.net*

Masaru Emoto: *www.masaru-emoto.net/english/e_ome_home.html.*

The Enneagram Institute: *www.enneagraminstitute.com*

Environmental Working Group: "Shopper's Guide to Pesticides": *www.foodnews.org/fulllist.php.*

Feng Shui: *www.fengshui.about.com*

Frank Ferrante: *May I Be Frank. www.mayibefrankmovie.com*

Fly Lady: *www.flylady.net*

Sean Foy: *The 10-Minute Total Body Breakthrough*. New York, NY: Workman Publishing Company, Inc., 2009.

David Heber, M.D., Ph.D.: *What Color Is Your Diet?* New York, NY: Harper Paperbacks, 2002.

Hay House: *www.hayhouse.com*

The Hoffman Institute International: *www.hoffmaninstitute.com*; "Negative Love," *A Path to Personal Freedom and Love,* www.hoffmaninstitute.org/process/path-to-personal-freedom/4.html

I Am a Miracle Foundation: *www.iamamiracle.com*

International Yang Family Tai Chi Chuan Association: *www.yangfamilytaichi.com/home*

Iyengar yoga: *www.iynaus.org*

Dr. Paul Jernigan: *www.divineloveheals.com*

Cheryl Karpen: *Eat Your Peas*. Anoka, MN: Gently Spoken, 2005.

Datis Kharrazian, D.H.Sc., D.C., M.S., M.NeuroSci: *Why Do I Still Have Thyroid Symptoms When My Lab Tests Are Normal: A Revolutionary Breakthrough In Understanding Hashimoto's Disease and Hypothyroidism*. Garden City, NY: Morgan James, 2010.

Fabrizio Mancini, D.C.: *The Power of Self-Healing: Unlock Your Natural Healing Potential in 21 Days!* Carlsbad, CA: Hay House, Inc., 2012

Tess Masters: *www.healthyblenderrecipes.com*

Mercola.com: Take Control of Your Health: *www.mercola.com*

Steve Meyerowitz: *Water – the Ultimate Cure: Discover Why Water Is the Most Important Ingredient in Your Diet and Find Out Which Water Is Right for You.* Great Barrington, MA: Sproutman Publications, 2000.

Mary Manin Morrissey: *www.marymorrissey.com*

Christiane Northrup, M.D.: *The Wisdom of Menopause: Creating Physical and Mental Health and Healing During the Change.* New York, NY: Bantam Dell, 2001.

Women's Bodies, Women's Wisdom: Creating Physical and Emotional Health and Healing. New York, NY: Bantam Dell, 2006. *www.drnorthrup.com*

James H. O'Keefe, M.D.: *The Forever Young Diet and Lifestyle.* Kansas City, MO: Andrews McMeel Publishing, 2006.

John O'Leary: *www.rising-above.com*

Mary Omwake: *www.maryomwake.com*

Rev. Joel Osteen: *www.joelosteen.com*

Mehmet Oz, M.D.: www.doctoroz.com

Rhythmic Medicine: *www.rhythmicmedicine.com*

Michelle Robin, D.C.: *Wellness on a Shoestring: Seven Habits for a Healthy Life.* Unity Village, MO: Unity Books, 2011. *www.drmichellerobin.com*

Suzanne M. Rowden, M.D.: *www.holisticfamilydoctorkc.com*

Jyotsna Sahni, M.D.: *www.drsahni.com*

Mark Stanton Welch: *www.markstantonwelch.com*

Sunlighten Infrared Saunas: *www.sunlightsaunas.com*

Jill Tupper: *www.jilltupper.com*

Unity: *www.unity.org*

Vitamix: *www.vitamix.com*

Your Wellness Connection: *www.yourwellnessconnection.com*

Dan Zarda: *Gratitude.* Seattle, WA: Compendium, 2010.

END NOTES

Chapter 1: Know Your Why

[1] Roger E. Bohn and James E. Short, "How Much Information? 2009 Report on American Consumers." December 2009. Global Information Industry Center, University of California San Diego.

Chapter 3: Plan Your Path

[1] Stephen R. Covey, *The 7 Habits of Highly Effective People* (New York, NY: Simon & Schuster, 1989).

[2] Michelle Robin, D.C., *Wellness on a Shoestring: Seven Habits for a Healthy Life* (Unity Village, MO: Unity Books, 2011).

Chapter 4: Find Your Tribe

[1] Seth Godin, *Tribes: We Need You to Lead Us* (New York, NY: Penguin Group, 2008).

[2] Abraham Maslow, "Maslow's Hierarchy of Needs." http://www.abraham-maslow.com/m_motivation/hierarchy_of_needs.asp (Accessed January 2012).

[3] Dan Buettner, *Blue Zones: Lessons for Living from the People Who've Lived the Longest* (Washington D.C.: National Geographic Society, 2008).

Chapter 6: Food As Fuel

[1,2,3] Woodson Merrell, M.D., *The Source: Unleash Your Natural Energy, Power Up Your Health and Feel 10 Years Younger* (New York, NY: Free Press, 2008).

[4] William Davis, M.D., *Wheat Belly: Lose the Wheat, Lose the Weight, and Find Your Path Back to Health* (New York, NY: Rodale, 2011).

Chapter 9: Relationship (As A Verb)

[1] Dan Buettner, *Blue Zones: Lessons for Living from the People Who've Lived the Longest* (Washington D.C.: National Geographic Society, 2008).

[2] May I Be Frank, www.mayibefrankmovie.com.

Chapter 10: Gratitude

[1] Morris Goodman, www.themiracleman.org.

Chapter 11: Service

[1] Gary Morsch, M.D. and Dean Nelson, *The Power of Serving Others: You Can Start Where You Are* (San Francisco, CA: Berrett-Koehler, 2006).

ACKNOWLEDGMENTS

Thank you, God, for giving me a passion for wellness and guiding me on this journey. I am humbled and honored to share my passion.

For all of you who have blessed me in my life and for taking time to love me, I am grateful.

To all my clients who have allowed me to care for you, for days or for years, you have touched my soul so deeply. Extra special thanks to Amy Gross, Joni Rogers, Jeanette Jayne, Karen Birdsall, Jodi Hobbs, Laura Henze, Marc Kaplan, and Jeanne Johnson for lovingly sharing your wellness journey.

To all my wonderful colleagues who continually share your gifts with the world: Sonia Choquette, John O'Leary, Dr. Fabrizio Mancini, Dr. Brooks Rice, Shelly Murray, Crystal Jenkins, Dr. Paul Jernigan, Dr. Jyotsna Sahni, Jill Tupper, Tess Masters, Frank Ferrante, and Dr. William Davis.

To my dear friend, Rebecca Korphage, thank you for all your support and for putting words to my voice.

To my editor, Betsy Stewart, thank you for your support and expertise.

To Shelly Murray, Shelly Gerber, Janet Vogt, and Debbie Garr for their extra support throughout manuscript development.

To all my team members at Your Wellness Connection, current and past, who have walked this journey with me: You will never know how grateful I am! You guys are amazing—every single day!

To all my coaches and mentors: Thank you, Ron and Linda Pfingsten, Dr. John and Carol Lakin, Dr. Richard Yennie, Pat Khan, Cindy Currie, Rev. Mary Omwake, Dr. Jack Sibley, Sally Smith, Bill and Vicki Reisler, Rev. Patricia Bass, Dr. Tom Hill, and Dr. Janice Hughes for loving me up, and continually sharing a wealth of guidance and wisdom.

To my colleagues at the Helzberg Entrepreneurial Mentoring Program, and especially to our fearless leader, Barnett Helzberg Jr., thank you for inspiring me.

To the greatest group of businesswomen in the universe—the *Kansas City Business Journal*'s "Women Who Mean Business"—thank you for pushing me to be the best I can be.

To my Translucent U Team—Cuky Harvey, Sonia Choquette, Karl and Kyle Peschke, Debra Graves, Mark Welch, Kimo, Brad Easton, Sabrina Tully and Crystal Jenkins—thank you for allowing me to grow in your sandbox.

To my family, thank you for all your love and support.

ABOUT THE AUTHOR

Michelle Robin, D.C. has been active in wellness for three decades. She is the author of the book *Wellness on a Shoestring: Seven Habits for a Healthy Life*, as well as a companion curriculum, *The Wellness on a Shoestring Program.* She is the founder of Your Wellness Connection, P.A., one of the nation's most successful healing centers focusing on integrative healing disciplines such as chiropractic, Chinese medicine, massage therapy, energy medicine, counseling, nutritional and wellness coaching, and movement arts.

Dr. Robin also assists businesses, non-profits, and faith-based communities in developing wellness programs. She shares her wellness message through local and national speaking engagements as well as collaborative efforts with other wellness practitioners and affiliates. Dr. Robin has spoken to a wide variety of groups including: Young Presidents Organization (YPO), AMC Theaters, Working Mother Magazine's Work Life Congress, Speaking of Women's Health Conference, Helzberg Entrepreneurial Mentoring Program, University of Kansas, University of Missouri-Kansas City, Unity Church (throughout the U.S.), and many others.

Dr. Robin holds a Bachelor of Business Administration degree from Washburn University and a Doctor of Chiropractic degree from Cleveland Chiropractic College. She has received post-graduate education from a number of institutions, including Parker College of Chiropractic, Logan College of Chiropractic, Cleveland Chiropractic College and Northwestern Health Sciences University.

The Masters Circle nationally recognized Dr. Robin as 2007 Chiropractor of the Year. Other awards include designation as one of the Kansas City Business Journal's "Women Who Mean Business" (2003); designation by the Kansas City Small Business Monthly as one of the "Top 25 under 25 Small Business" (2002); and the House of Menuha Community Service Award (2005). Most recently Dr. Robin received the Speaking of Women's Health "Glow" award (2010) and the eWomen Network Femtor "Made it to a Million" Award (2011). She is a regular contributing writer to various community publications.

As an active member of the community, Dr. Robin has held a variety of non-profit board positions including: HEMP, KC Free Health Clinic,

SAFEHOME, Menorah Legacy Foundation, Turning Point, as well as served on committees for WIN For KC, Speaking of Women's Health, HEMP, House of Menuha, and Go Red for Women.